Clean Eating is Eating Clean

A Proven Step-by-Step Guide to Eating Clean From Home Recipes to On-the-go Fast Food Options

Introduction

Clean Eating occupies a unique place among the many diets available today. More than a diet, it is a lifestyle that allows for healthy eating without sacrificing flavor and taste. Aside from its variety of benefits, ranging from weight loss, protection from health risks to savings on finances, Clean Eating is becoming the preferred choice.

This guide presents you with the basics of Clean Eating, the recommended food groups, the minimization or avoidance of processed food and core principles that can guide you on this lifestyle.

Plus, it shows you a comparison between the cost of eating out and cooking in both in terms of financial and nutritional value. There is also a grocery guide to help you when you shop for Clean Eating-friendly items. Also, since fast foods and restaurants may not be fully avoided, a guide on how to retain the lifestyle when you find yourself with no other options is also included.

Clean Eating recipes, for breakfast, lunch, dinner and snacks are also included to help you jumpstart your first days on the Clean Eating lifestyle.

Table of Contents

Step One: Discover Clean Eating

Clean Eating is beginning to gain not only popularity but also recognition. With support from various health experts, personal trainers and celebrity endorsers, Clean Eating has become the choice for achieving the desired and ideal status of health and well-being. Among the many diet fads and trends, Clean Eating occupies unique and refreshing recommendations for the way we eat.

Unlike many diets, Clean Eating's claim to fame is because it is not a diet at all. In fact, it is an overall lifestyle choice that is very inclusive, flexible and friendly to both health and taste. While other diets give absolute restrictions Clean Eating except for one rule, allows tolerance. While other diets are rigid in their proportions and ingredients, Clean Eating is more lenient. While other diets are unforgiving of failure, Clean Eating is open to changes and creativity.

Below are the five guiding principles of Clean Eating:

1. Choose whole and natural instead of refined and processed.

2. Include protein, fat and carbohydrate and minimize salt and sugar

3. Eat, not drink, calories

4. Consume five to six small instead of two to three large meals

5. Drink water

However, Clean Eating does not mean complete freedom from eating anything that you want. To access the wide range of benefits that Clean Eating can provide, there are certain food items that must be avoided. Clean Eating does not allow for ultra- processed foods or additives in the meals.

Below is a list of ideas that can help you identify processed food:

1. Canned, boxed, bagged or packaged, they are considered processed, except of course for a bag of vegetables.

2. Preserved, these are items with high content of salt to let them keep for long periods of time.

3. Flavored, sugar is added to these food items to make them more appealing to the taste and more addictive.

4. Enriched, although seeing labels that claim to have infused the product with vitamins and other essential nutrients, these are still counted as processed because they add something that is not naturally there in the first place.

5. Manufactured, these are entire food items that are not naturally occurring at all but are created in a laboratory or a factory.

Remember, processed food does not automatically make them bad for you. For example, canning out of season fruits so we can still buy them the entire year is good. Some processing, such as milk, is done to remove bacteria or toxins that are dangerous for human consumption. Blending vegetables, fruits and other ingredients, such as smoothies, to make them easier to digest is still good but technically still processed.

The main principle of Clean Eating is proper portioning. Your best effort must always be geared towards consuming the best, most natural and healthiest version of the food items that you can access. It will be perfect if you can completely avoid all processed food, however due to the current technology and food preparation trends today, it may be difficult to completely abstain from processed food. Your best option is to limit your intake of processed foods.

Step Two: Gain the Benefits of the Lifestyle

Clean Eating is usually associated with producing a variety of benefits that are highly desirable, not only because of their holistic impact to health but also because of practical and more popular advantages.

Some of the benefits of Clean Eating are:

1. Weight loss

2. More energy & better sleep

3. More youthful skin & shinier hair

4. Improved mental faculties

5. Prevention and protection from risks and diseases

Due to the proper portioning recommended by Clean Eating, you are in a better position to control your weight. Consuming high calorie food types that are beyond what your body needs will only be stored as fat in your bodies. This unnecessary reserve of energy is dangerous because it opens you to risks from hypertension, diabetes and cardiovascular diseases. With the proper intake of calories, your consumption and use of calories are well-balanced.

Aside from the prevention of the accumulation of fats through unused calories, Clean Eating gives you sustained energy the entire day. You can avoid peaks or bursts provided by large meals and the corresponding crash time when the effects of the sugar high die down. Aside from that, when you taper off the consumption of sugar, you can have a more relaxing and restful sleep that can energize you for the next day.

Another effect of Clean Eating is on the skin. When you eliminate toxins in your body you can reduce breakouts, acne and other skin conditions. When you increase intake of naturally occurring vitamins such as A, C and E in the food groups recommended by Clean Eating, your skin heals faster, becomes more elastic and smoother. Since hair is technically part of the same body system as skin, it becomes shinier, less brittle and more manageable.

With your body infused with relatively the exact and timely amounts of nutrients it needs, the mind also improves. Your quick thinking produces better results, memory is enhanced and a general positive outlook in life is developed.

Aside from these benefits, with Clean Eating, you are beginning to reduce the risks your body may have from illnesses and diseases. As you reduce the fat you store, you can begin to clear and dissolve unwanted deposits on your arteries or blood vessels. With sugar down, you reduce the risk for diabetes. With salt intake at a minimum, hypertension and the diseases associated with it are also reduced.

Step Three: Compare the Costs of Eating Out & Cooking In

Another bonus benefit of Clean Eating is on the finances. Aside from the many positive health consequences of this lifestyle, you can actually either save on expenses or get more nutrition for the same price.

Most fast food or restaurant meals are prepared and served to you with almost none to minimal control from your end. This means that even if you plan to follow the Clean Eating lifestyle, you may unwittingly fail it when you eat out. Generally, eating out involves meals that are filled with sugar, salt and fats due to its preparation. Unless you are dining in a very Clean Eating-friendly restaurant, chances are, the food will have more than one processed ingredient.

There are two cases where traditional grocery is a better alternative, first in terms of monetary value and second in terms of nutritional value. For the first case, take for example a steak, soup and salad meal. On an average steak restaurant, the cost for one serving will be $20 for the steak, $5 for the soup and $5 for the salad. Total for the meal is $30; add tariff, taxes, service charge or tip, the final bill will be around $40.

Next to recreate the actual meal, $7 for the vegetables, $4 for the soup and $20 for a pound of steak and another $5 for miscellaneous cooking items. Total bill is $36. Compare the total restaurant bill of $40 and $36 for the groceries, the $4 may seem too small of a margin to convince someone to cook at home instead of eating out. However, take note the $36 is actually good for around 3 to 4 servings of the entire meal. The actual cost per person per meal, complete with the steak, the soup and the salad will be from $9 to $12. Now compare $9 grocery to the $40 restaurant bill, this represents a $31 savings.

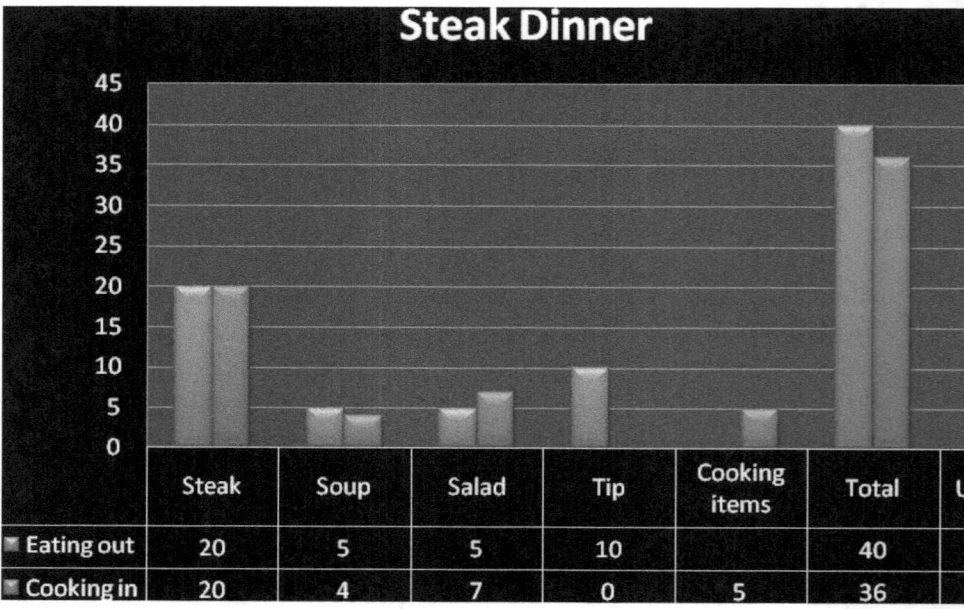

Steak Dinner

	Steak	Soup	Salad	Tip	Cooking items	Total
Eating out	20	5	5	10		40
Cooking in	20	4	7	0	5	36

For the second case, you can spend the same amount on a fast food or on a box of processed food and on grocery items. For relatively the same price, you can actually get rid of processed foods and choose Clean Eating-friendly ingredients.

For $20, you can buy 8 pieces of fried chicken, 4 pieces of biscuits, 1 side of mashed potato and 1 side of corn at a popular chicken fast food chain. To recreate a Clean Eating version of the same meal, you can buy 2 lbs. of chicken breasts for $1.95, 10 lbs. of potatoes for $3 and 8 ears of corn for $2. Total grocery bill should now be at around $7. With $13 more to spare, you can buy 1 tub of yogurt for $3, various legumes and vegetables for a salad for $5, 1 gallon of milk for $2 and 1 lb. of lean beef for $3 for an additional course.

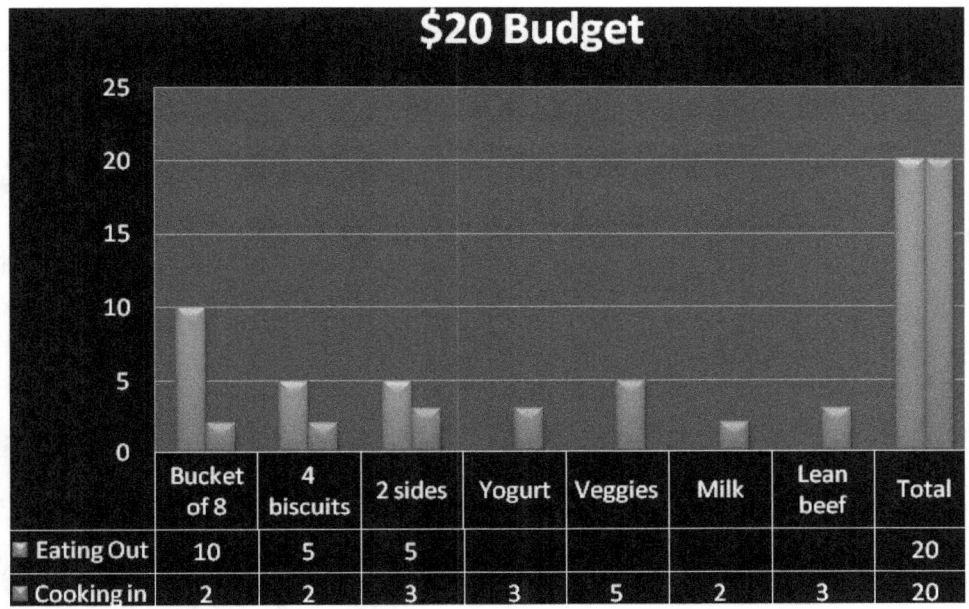

	Bucket of 8	4 biscuits	2 sides	Yogurt	Veggies	Milk	Lean beef	Total
Eating Out	10	5	5					20
Cooking in	2	2	3	3	5	2	3	20

Step Four: Shop at the Grocery for Clean Foods

When you begin to shift your eating lifestyle away from eating out to cooking in or choosing to buy your own ingredients and prepare your own meals, it will be important to become a savvy buyer in the grocery. Unless you are buying in a specialty grocery that commits to Clean Eating-friendly merchandise, you have to be very careful when you are buying.

If it is your first time in buying your groceries for a Clean Eating lifestyle, it may be hard at first. You may find yourself confused, roaming around the aisles or taking a long time to scrutinize every product on the shelf. However, as you develop your familiarity with the grocery items, you can begin to have your own go-to brands, packages or entire sections. Buying Clean Eating-friendly ingredients will soon become second nature to you and buying groceries will be a breeze.

Here are few recommendations to help you come up with a grocery list, they are meant to help you not only to increase nutritional value but also minimize cost and exposure to processed foods:

1. Learn about the seasonal vegetables and fruits. When they are in season, they are fresher and cheaper in the grocery.

2. Whether vegetable or fruit, buying whole is better than pre-cut. They cost less and the nutrients are still intact because the skin is still untouched.

3. The brighter the better. For vegetables and fruits, if you are choosing between two packages of carrots, choose the more vivid color, it has more phytochemicals. They have more antioxidants and vitamins are intact.

4. Avoid whites. White sugar, white flour, white bread, white rice and other white products are meant to look clean to make them more appealing to buyers. However, these items undergo lengthy processing times before they end up with the white color they have. Often, aside from losing the nutrients they originally had, these items also have harmful additives.

5. Less is more. The fewer ingredients in a meal or the fewer components in a food item, the better it is and the more Clean-Eating friendly it becomes. You can use this principle to guide you especially when you are down to 2 items in a grocery and you are comparing which one is better.

6. Deconstruct a ready-to-eat meal. Instead of choosing a packaged version of a grocery item, try to break it down to its naturally occurring components. For example, instead of buying a carton of orange juice, the basic ingredient is oranges. Either buy a pack of oranges or have them bottle a freshly squeezed version of it.

Here is a tentative list of grocery items that you can refer to when you are planning to restock your kitchen or pantry. For some reason, they are mostly found on the outer perimeters of the grocery, while the inner aisles and shelves are filled with processed foods.

1. Brown rice

2. Black, pinto or cannellini beans and chickpeas

3. Raw almonds, walnuts or cashews

4. Lettuce, garlic, tomatoes, onions, kale, parsley, broccoli, brussels sprouts or any vegetable that you like

5. Organic and free range proteins are preferred over packaged meats, chicken breast, salmon, tuna, lean meats, tilapia and shrimp

6. Coconut, sesame or extra virgin olive oil

7. Black pepper, cayenne, cinnamon, tamari, Dijon mustard, apple cider or red wine vinegar, basil, oregano and rosemary

8. Grapes, berries, lemons, avocado, apples, bananas or any fruit that you like

9. Teas, coconut water or freshly squeezed fruits for beverages and honey to sweeten

Step Five: Stay Safe at the Fast Food

In an ideal world, you will always have access or options to choose Clean Eating over processed food. However, the reality is you will find yourself in a situation where a fast food or a restaurant is your only option for your meals. Try as you may, you may never avoid them. Instead of giving in to temptation, you can be more mindful of your choices even within these establishments and you can do your best to minimize your exposure to processed foods.

Here are some tips to help you make the best choice in the menu when you are eating out in a fast food:

1. Choose a veggie o a turkey version of the burger; substitute the mayonnaise with pickles or ask to hold it entirely. Ask for a whole-wheat version of the bread when available. For example, choose the Burger King: Veggie Burger

2. Ask for water instead of the beverages. Most of the time the fruit juices are only from powder or concentrates. For example, Lemonades are always made from powder.

3. Most fast food comes in a complete package of a main course, a side and a soda. Eat only half of the main and take the whole side dish if it is vegetables and skip the soda. For example, McDonald's Southwest Salad and Oatmeal are good alternatives to its meals.

4. Choose soft instead of the hard or fried tacos when possible. For example, Taco Bell's Soft Tacos are better than its fried tortilla versions. Instead of beef, ask for chicken or bean tacos.

5. When you order, find out which of the menu has the least number of ingredients. When you order salad,

make sure to ask the waiter to hold the bread, cheese and dressing.

6. When you order Chinese food, ask for brown rice and steamed vegetables.

7. Choose sashimi or nigiri when eating at a Japanese restaurant, often the more complicated the sushi, the more additives are in it.

Step Six: Prepare for the Lifestyle

Although there is no better time to start with the Clean Eating lifestyle than today, it is best to prepare yourself and your environment for it. It may be better to postpone your start to give way for adequate preparation instead of starting haphazardly and risk failing.

Here are some tips to help you with Day Zero or the timeframe before the actual start of your Clean Eating lifestyle:

1. Adjust yourself by making gradual changes to your eating habits. Instead of making a complete turnaround, start with minor substitutes. Instead of white bread for breakfast, you may opt to choose the whole-wheat version. Instead of a chocolate bar for snacks, try a pack of fruit varieties. Instead of a soda for drinks, choose a fruit juice.

2. Set your health goals. Formulate your goal statement in a SMART way. This acronym stands for specific, measurable, attainable, relevant and time-bound. The smarter your goal is, the better you can monitor your progress and motivate you to success.

3. Measure your baseline health statistics. Take your weight, blood pressure, blood sugar levels or other information so you have an idea of the figures prior to your Clean Eating lifestyle. Track improvements as you go along with the meals.

4. Check your kitchen and pantry. Make sure to remove or dispose any processed food or non-Clean Eating friendly food items. This will either protect you from unknowingly using these items when you cook at home or from giving into temptation.

5. If you are sharing your home with your family or friends, it is important to inform them of your plans to adopt a Clean Eating lifestyle. They will be able to support you when you introduce the new meal plans to them. If possible, ask them to join you on your plans.

Step Seven: Cook the Meals

5 Breakfasts

Title: Egg Skillet- a healthy and tasty breakfast to start your day. The oregano and pepper flakes will give you that added jolt that can wake you for an early start.

Servings: 4

Ingredients:

1 tbsp olive oil

1 thinly sliced white onion

3 cloves minced garlic

½ tsp dried oregano

4 cups chopped spinach

4 cups chopped collard greens

5 sliced white mushrooms

4 large eggs

2 tbsp Greek yogurt

1 tbsp milk

½ tsp pepper flakes

¼ tsp sea salt

Pepper to taste

Directions:

Preheat oven to 400 degrees

Using a pot, heat oil on medium to high and add salt, pepper and collard greens.

Stir until vegetables become radiant green or for about 3 minutes

Add garlic, oregano and pepper flakes. Stir.

Add spinach and stir for 2 minutes. Remove heat.

Remove mixture and place in skillet. Garnish with mushrooms.

Make 4 wells in the mixture and crack eggs into the wells.

Bake for 8 to 10 minutes

In a separate bowl, whisk milk, yogurt and 1 clove of garlic.

Spread mixture on top of spinach mixture.

Serve.

Picture:

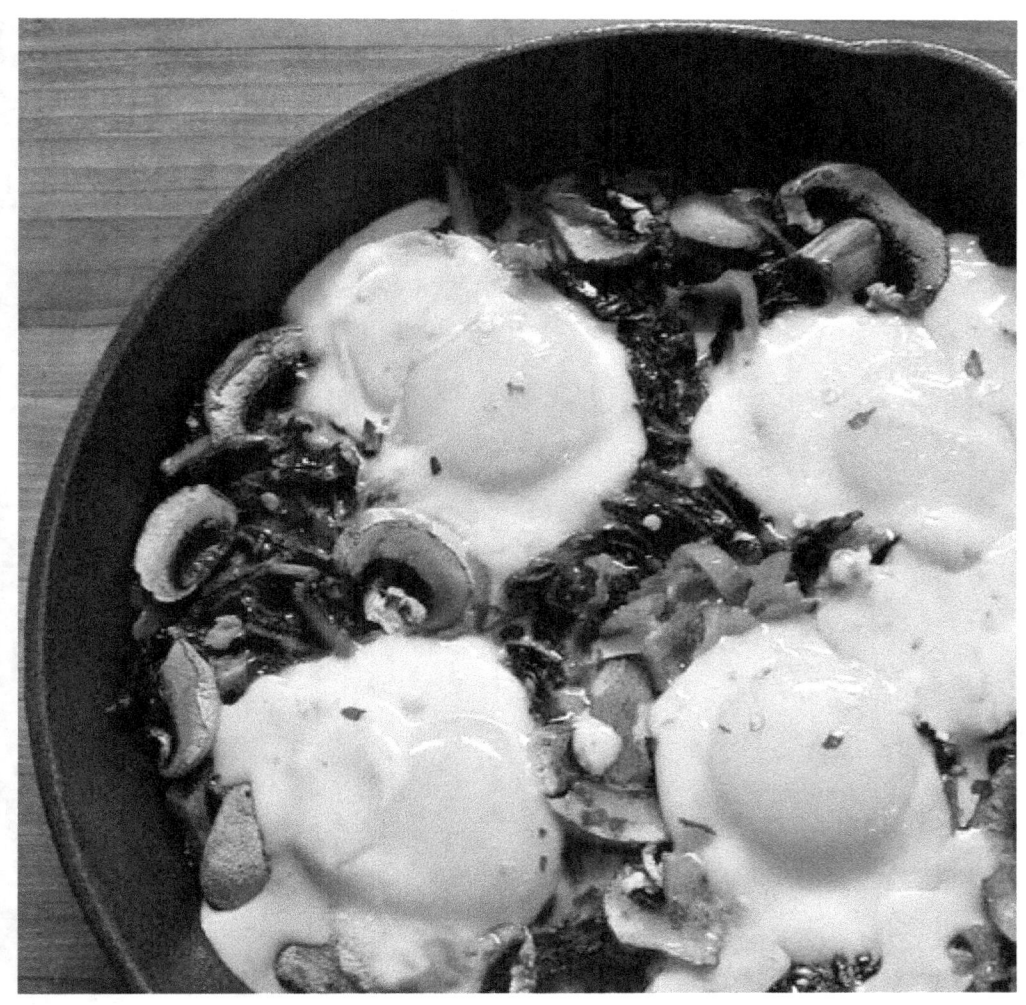

Nutritional Value:

Calories: 150

Total fat: 9g

Saturated fat: 2g

Carbs: 8g

Fiber: 3g

Sugar: 3g

Protein: 10g

Sodium: 281 mg

Cholesterol: 212 mg

Title: Breakfast Rice Bowl- a simple breakfast that will give you the traditional flavors of a sweet breakfast without the sugar additives that can only amplify your sugar addiction.

Servings: 4

Ingredients:

1 cup halved dark cherries

1 cup brown rice

2 tsp ground cinnamon

½ tsp orange zest

¼ cup skim milk

¼ tsp sea salt

½ tsp vanilla extract

4 tsp maple syrup

Directions:

Cook rice

In a bowl, combine rice, cinnamon, zest and salt. Divide mixture into 4 bowls

In a saucepan, boil milk and syrup on medium heat. Remove heat and add vanilla. Drizzle on top of mixture and top with cherries.

Serve.

Picture:

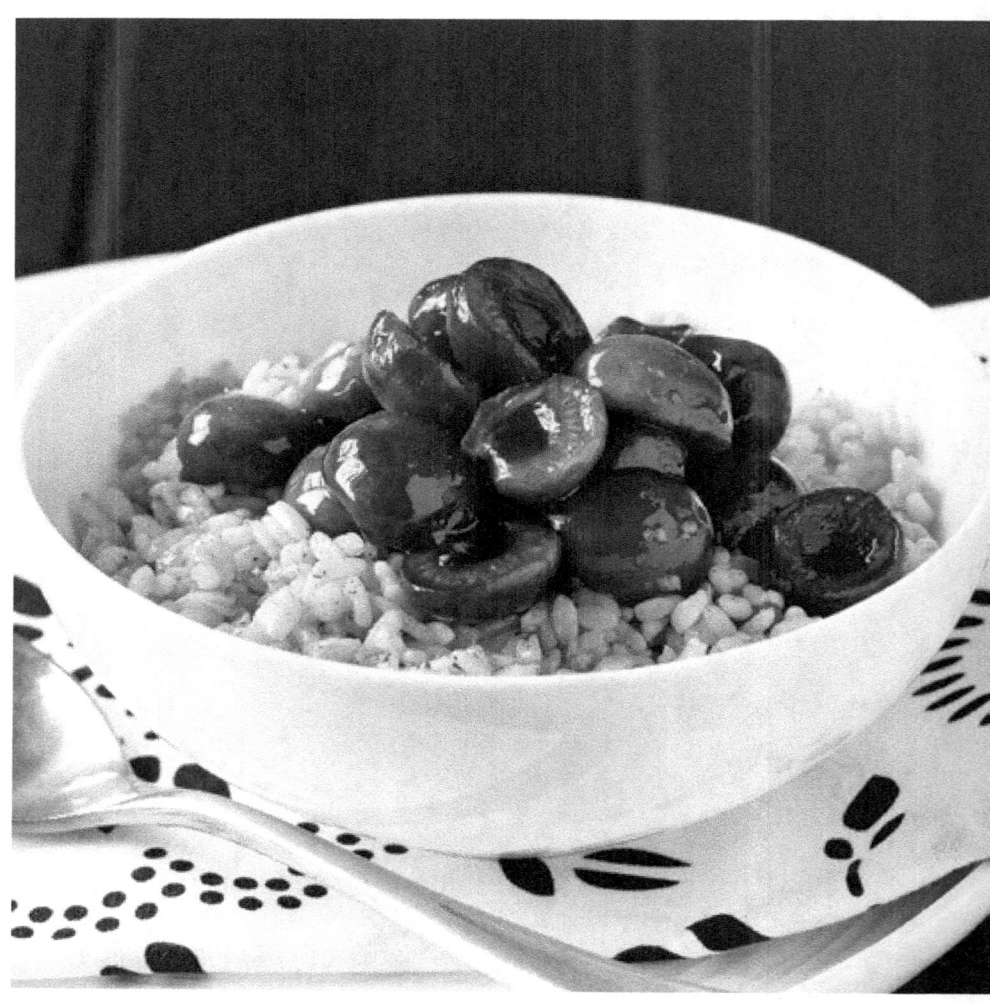

Nutritional Value:

Calories: 253

Total fat: 5 g

Sat. fat: 0.5g

Monounsaturated fat: 3g

Polyunsaturated fat: 1g

Carbs: 48g

Fiber: 4g

Sugar: 9g

Protein: 5g

Sodium: 136mg

Cholesterol: 0mg

Title: Citrus Salad- a citrus-based breakfast for the person on-the-go, it is easy to prepare and full of flavors and textures at the same time.

Servings: 4

Ingredients:

1 orange

1 grapefruit

2 mandarin oranges

1 Jamaican tangelo

4 kumquats

2 tbsp chopped mint leaves

Directions:

Peel skin of fruits and pull apart. Cut into bite sized pieces

Add kumquats and mint.

Toss and refrigerate for 15 minutes

Picture:

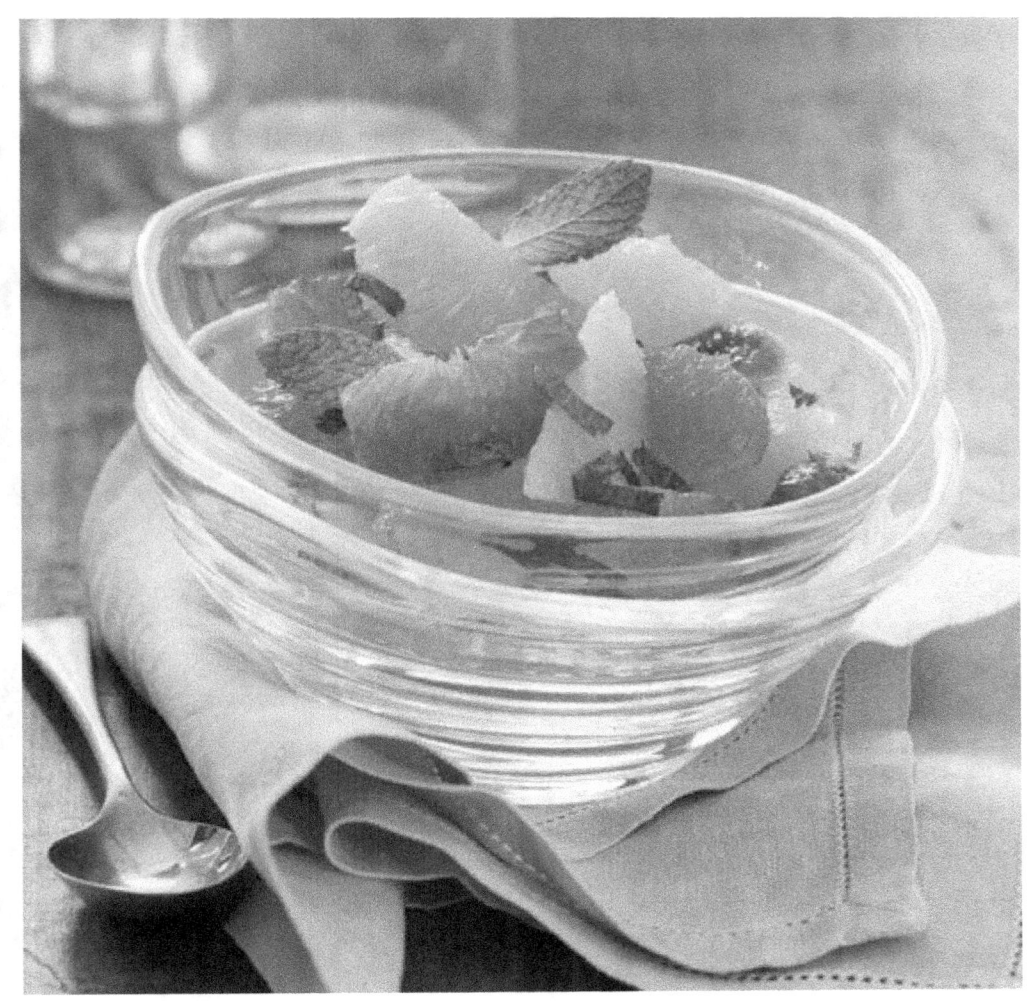

Nutritional Value:

Calories: 148

Total fat: 0.2g

Sat. fat: 0.1g

Carbs: 36g

Fiber: 5g

Protein: 2g

Sodium: 9mg

Cholesterol: 0mg

Title: Breakfast Cocktail- a breakfast that you can store on a tumbler and take on your way to school or work, it is great for the summer and can also be refreshment during the afternoon

Servings: 1

Ingredients:

2 stalks celery

2 oz spinach

1 cored tomato

½ peeled lemon

Directions:

Using a juicer, start with the celery, spinach, tomato then lemon.

Stir and serve with ice

Picture:

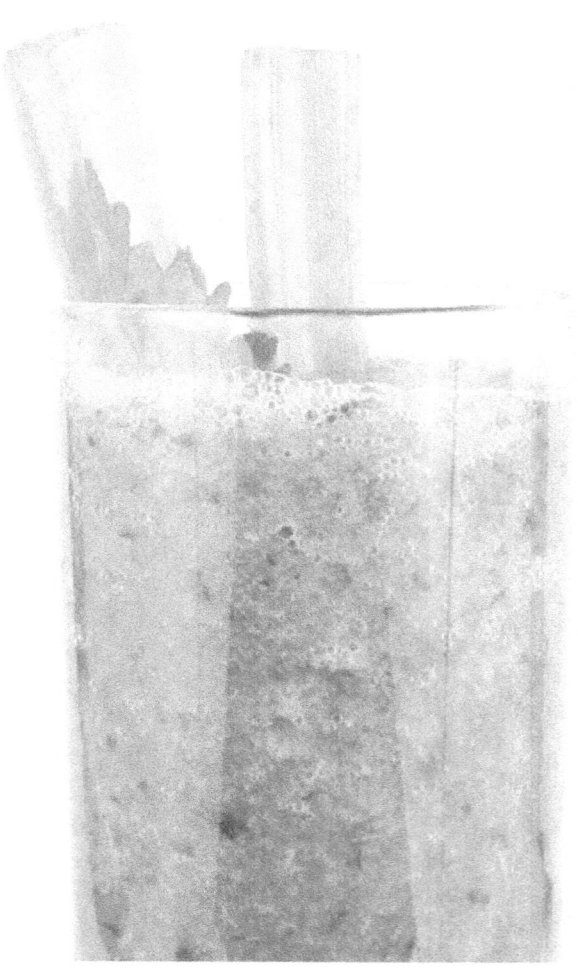

Nutritional Value:

Calories: 64

Total fat: 0g

Fat: 0g

Carbs: 16g

Fiber: 6g

Sugar: 6g

Protein: 2g

Sodium: 202mg

Cholesterol: 0mg

Title: Veggie Hash- a money-saver alternative for breakfast that can make use of leftovers from veggie dinners, it is easy to cook, pleasant to the eyes and delicious to the taste.

Servings: 6

Ingredients:

1 acorn squash, peeled and cut into ¼ inch pieces

¾ lb small potatoes

Olive oil spray

4 tsp olive oil

2 minced shallots

2 cups shredded broccoli

1/3 cup red bell pepper thinly sliced

1/3 cup green bell pepper thinly sliced

2 tsp lemon juice

½ tsp sea salt

½ tsp black pepper

Directions:

Heat oven to 425 degrees

In a separate bowl, toss potatoes and squash with salt and pepper

Spray oil on baking sheet and place mixture

Drizzle with oil and toss

Bake until tender or for 25 minutes.

Stir occasionally

Heat oil in skillet on medium to high

Sauté bell peppers, broccoli and shallots

Add mixture and cook for 5 minutes

Drizzle with lemon juice and salt and pepper to taste

Serve

Picture:

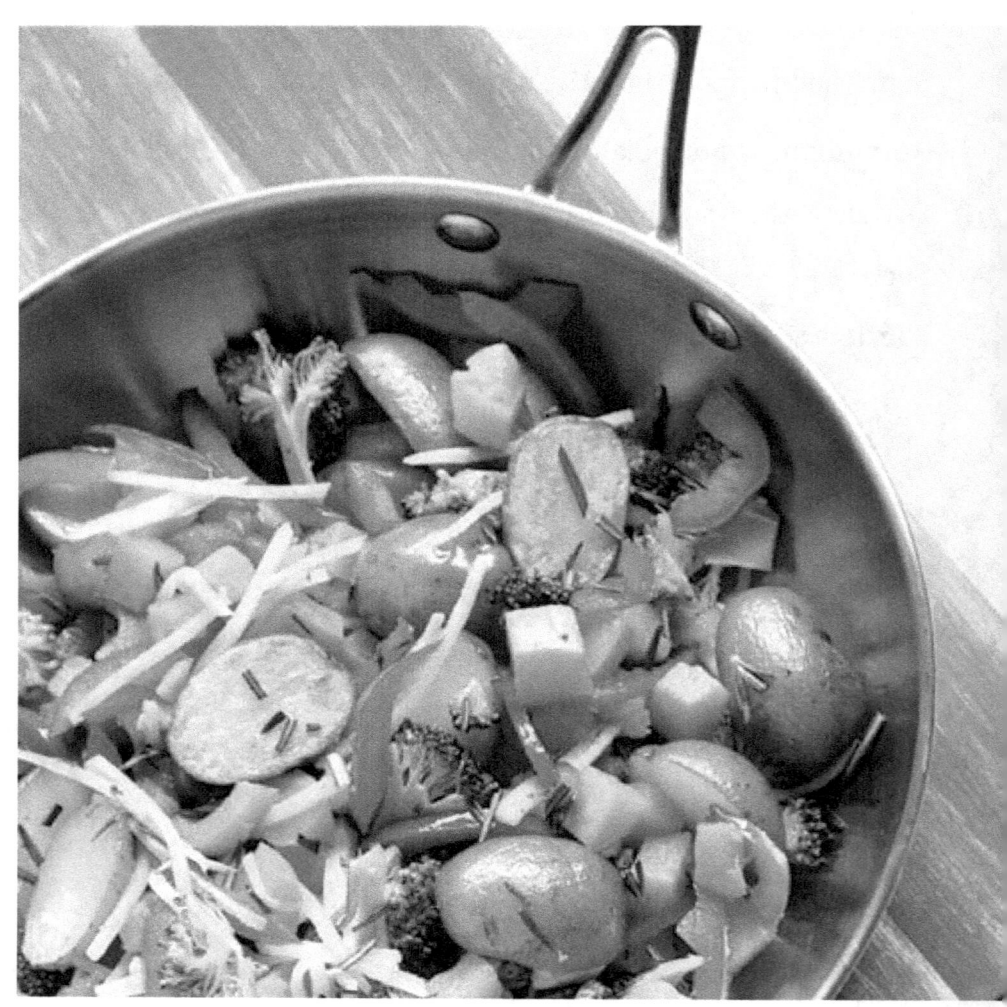

Nutritional Value:

Calories: 120

Total fat: 3g

Sat. fat: 0g

Carbs: 21g

Fiber: 3g

Sugar: 3g

Protein: 3.5g

Sodium: 170mg

Cholesterol: 0mg

10 Lunches

Title: Spinach Sandwich- a quick lunch that you can easily pack to the office. Easy to eat at the same time without the mess and cleanup needed.

Servings: 4

Ingredients:

1 cup spinach

4 slices whole grain bread

2 pears, peeled, cored, seeded and sliced in ½ inch

2 tsp canola oil

1 tsp lemon juice

Directions:

Heat oven to 400 degrees

In a separate bowl, whisk oil, juice and pear

Place in baking sheet and roast for 20 minutes

Toast bread and top with mixture

Press bread together

Serve

Picture:

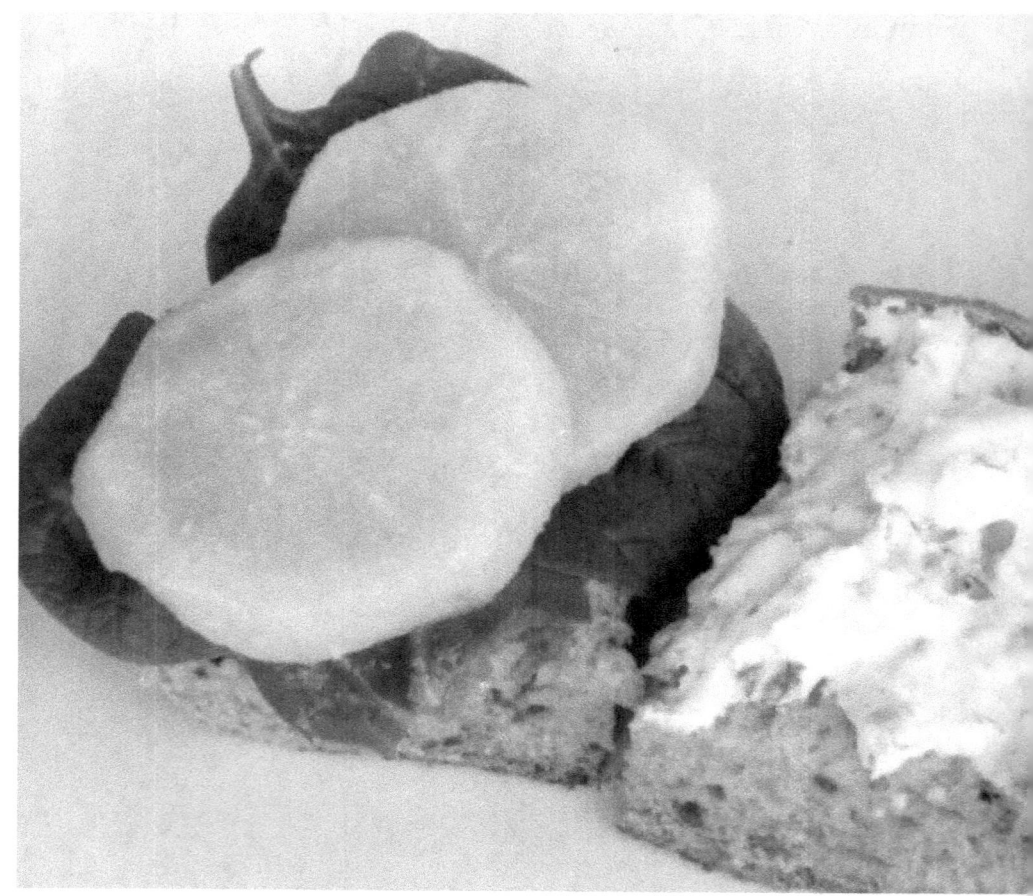

Nutritional Value:

Calories: 176

Total fat: 6 g

Sat. fat: 2g

Trans fat: 0g

Cholesterol: 5mg

Sodium: 159 mg

Carbs: 26g

Fiber: 5g

Sugar: 11g

Protein: 6g

Title: Cobb Salad- a colorful lunch that is packed with flavors, from sweet avocados and tomatoes to the acid of the dressing and vegetables.

Servings: 6

Ingredients:

2 eggs, boiled, peeled and sliced

6 cup chopped lettuce

2 avocadoes, peeled, seeded and sliced into 1 inch pieces

1 chicken breast, cooked, skinned and cubed

2 chopped tomatoes

For the dressing: ¼ cup vinegar, ½ cup extra virgin olive oil, 1 tsp honey and salt and pepper to taste

Directions:

Toss all ingredients in a large bowl.

Picture:

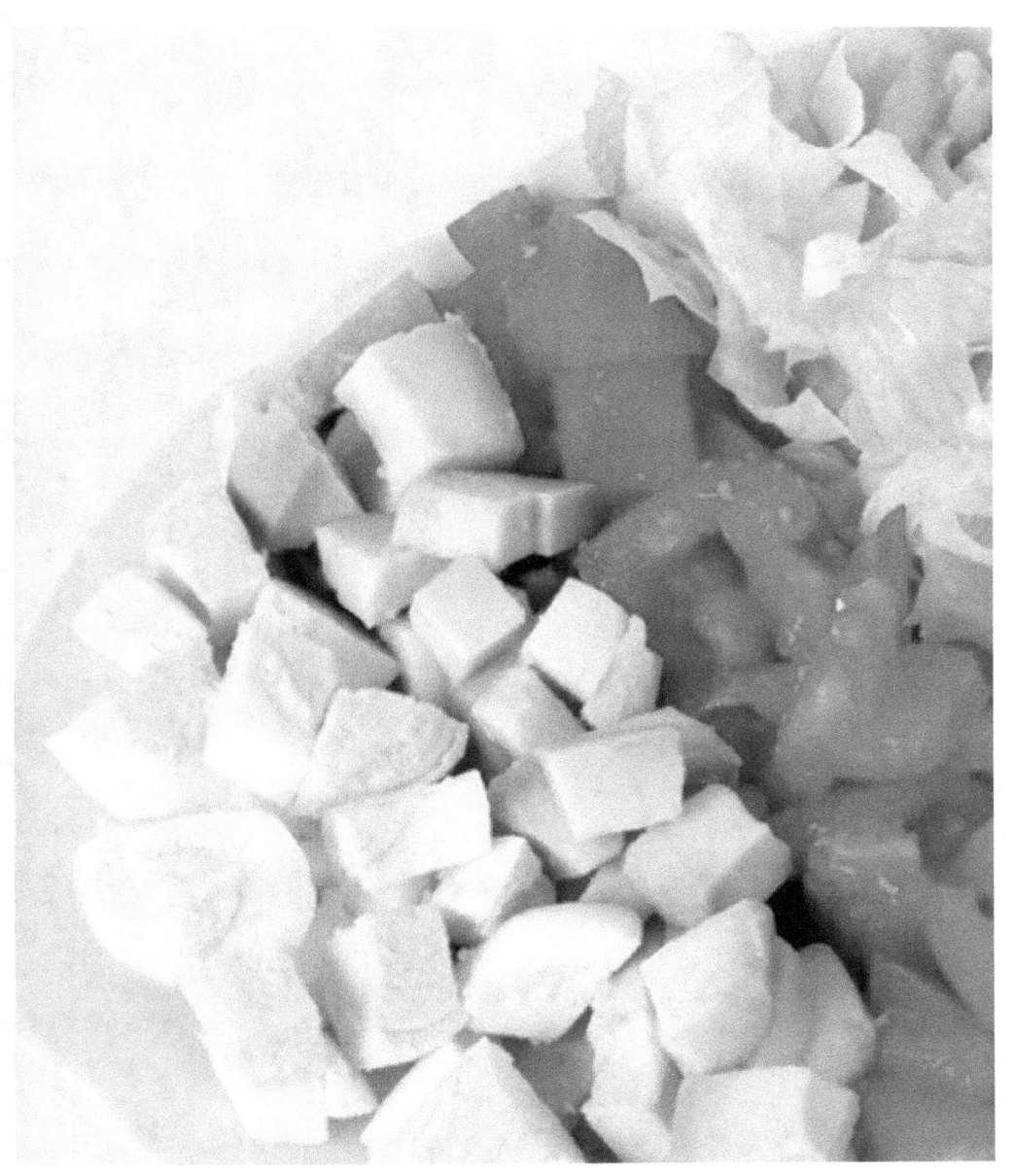

Nutritional Value:

Calories: 282

Total fat: 24g

Sat. fat: 4g

Trans fat: 0g

Cholesterol: 84g

Carbs: 8g

Sodium: 437 mg

Fiber: 4g

Sugar: 4g

Protein: 10g

Title: Burrito Wrap- a healthy version of a popular meal retains the taste as with the original but with natural nutrients from its healthy ingredients, it is great for a long work day.

Servings: 6

Ingredients:

6 cups spinach finely chopped

15 oz. black beans

1.5 cup brown rice

½ cup chopped lettuce

½ cup reduced fat cheese, grated

½ cup salsa

6 tbsp Greek yogurt

6 whole grain wraps

Salt and pepper to taste

Directions:

Heat oven to 300 degrees

Wrap stacked tortillas in foil

Put on baking sheet and bake for 15 minutes

Use skillet and heat to medium

Put beans and spinach and heat for 3 minutes

Put mixture in wraps

Add ¼ cup of rice on each wrap

Add lettuce, salsa, yogurt, cheese lettuce

Fold and serve

Picture:

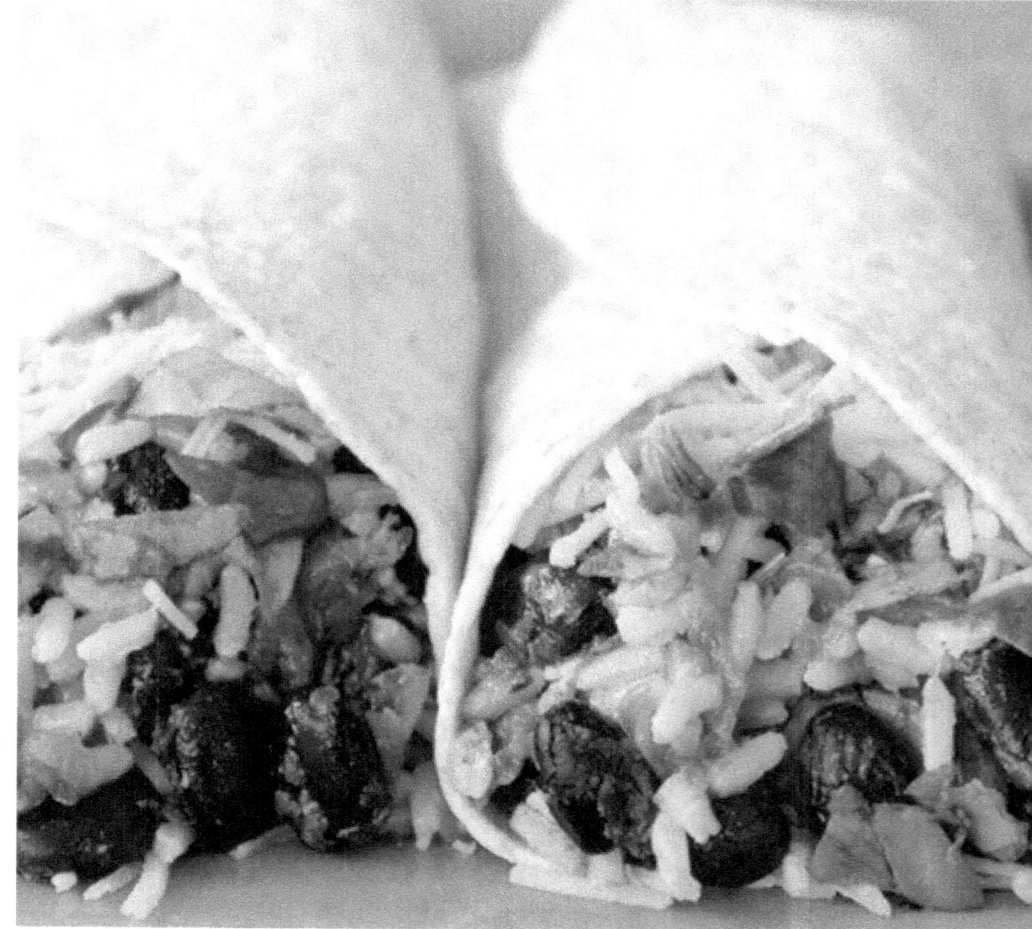

Nutritional Value:

Calories: 282

Total fat: 5g

Sat. fat: 1g

Trans fat: 0g

Cholesterol: 3g

Carbs: 50g

Sodium: 560mg

Fiber: 5g

Sugar: 3g

Protein: 13g

Title: Quinoa Salad- a adventurous lunch for the veteran Clean Eater, its texture add excitement to the already flavorful meal.

Servings: 6

Ingredients:

1 cup rinsed quinoa

1 cup garbanzo beans

1 tomato, chopped

1 cucumber, chopped

2 cloves garlic, diced

10 small basil leaves, sliced

1 tsp grated ginger

1 lemon, juiced

2 small carrots, diced

1 cup low fat cheese

Salt and pepper, extra virgin oil and balsamic vinegar

Directions:

Toss all ingredients in large bowl

Refrigerate for 30 minutes

Serve

Picture:

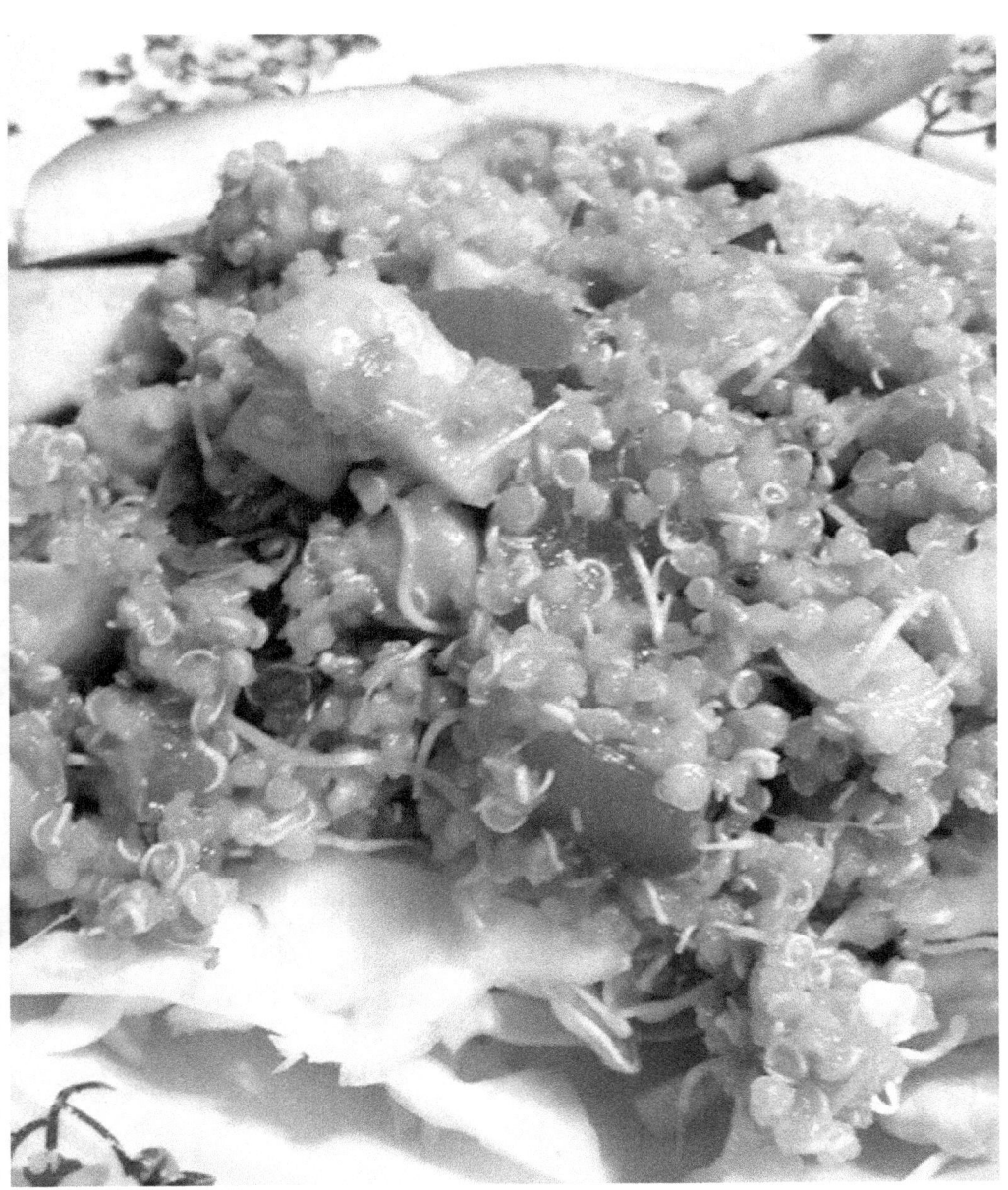

Nutritional Value:

Calories: 259

Total fat: 5g

Sat. fat: 2gm

Trans fat: 0gm

Cholesterol: 4mg

Sodium: 436mg

Carbs: 40g

Fiber: 9g

Sugar: 4g

Protein: 12g

Title: Chicken & Berry Salad- a heavy lunch for a busy day, combine a variety of textures from the smooth chicken, the crunchy almonds and the tasty berries

Servings: 4

Ingredients:

2 cups cubed and cooked chicken breasts

1 cup blueberries

5 cups mixed green vegetables

¼ cup almonds

For the dressing: ¼ cup olive oil, ¼ cup blueberries, 2tbsp honey, ¼ cup apple cider vinegar and salt and pepper

Directions:

In a large bowl, toss all ingredients

In a separate bowl, combine all dressing ingredients and put in a blender.

Blend till smooth

Add salt and pepper

Serve

Picture:

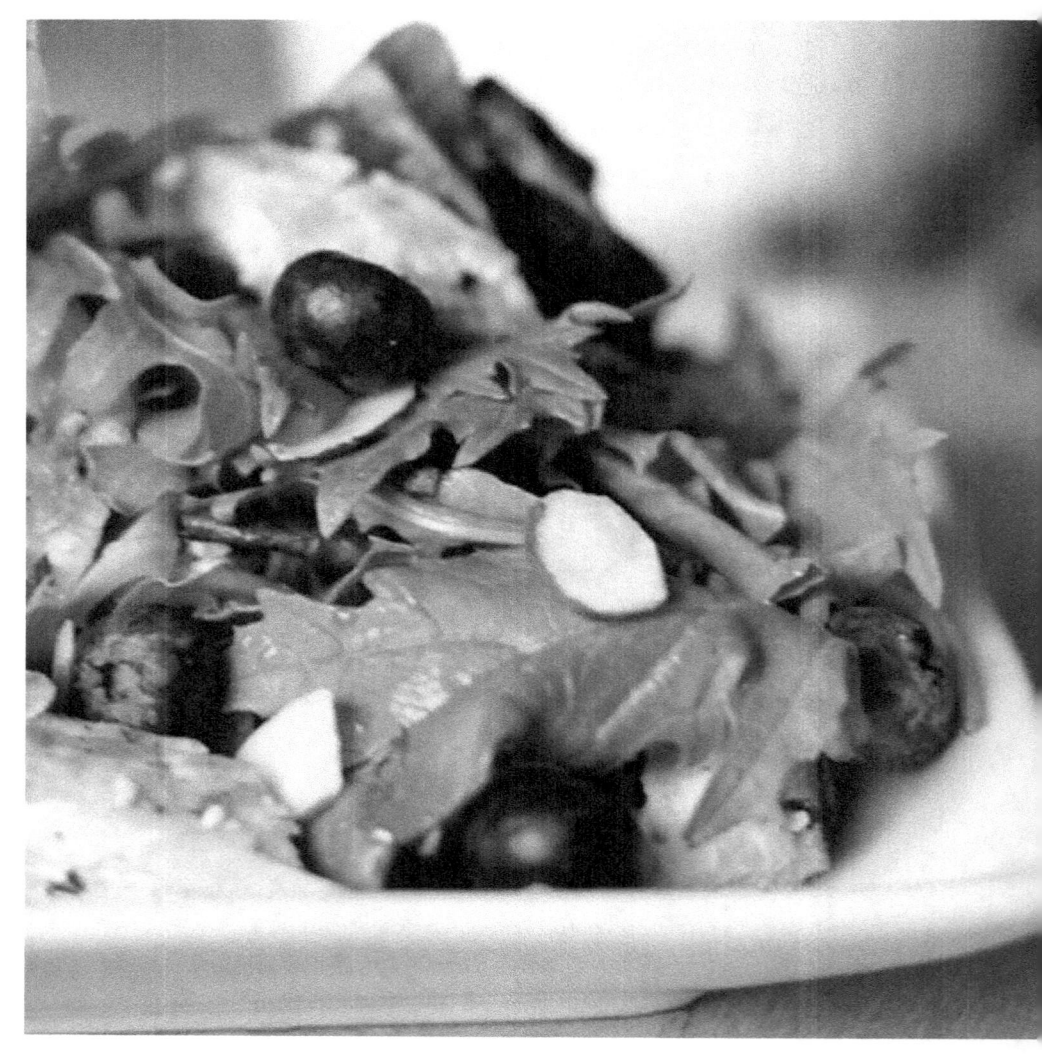

Nutritional Value:

Calories: 266

Total fat: 18g

Sat. fat: 3g

Cholesterol: 25mg

Sodium: 60mg

Carbs: 18g

Fiber: 3g

Sugar: 14g

Protein: 11g

Title: Pears and Feta Mix- a surprising twist to the otherwise unassuming pear, it is pleasing to the eye, tongue and health.

Servings: 4

Ingredients:

8 cup spring mix

1 red onion, halved

2 tbsp olive oil

2 medium pears, peeled, seeded and sliced into wedges

½ cup fat-free feta cheese

Directions:

Heat oven to 400 degrees

Combine pear with oil and place on baking sheet

Roast each side for 10 minutes, allow cooling

Toss rest of ingredients in a salad bowl

Sprinkle with cheese

Serve

Picture:

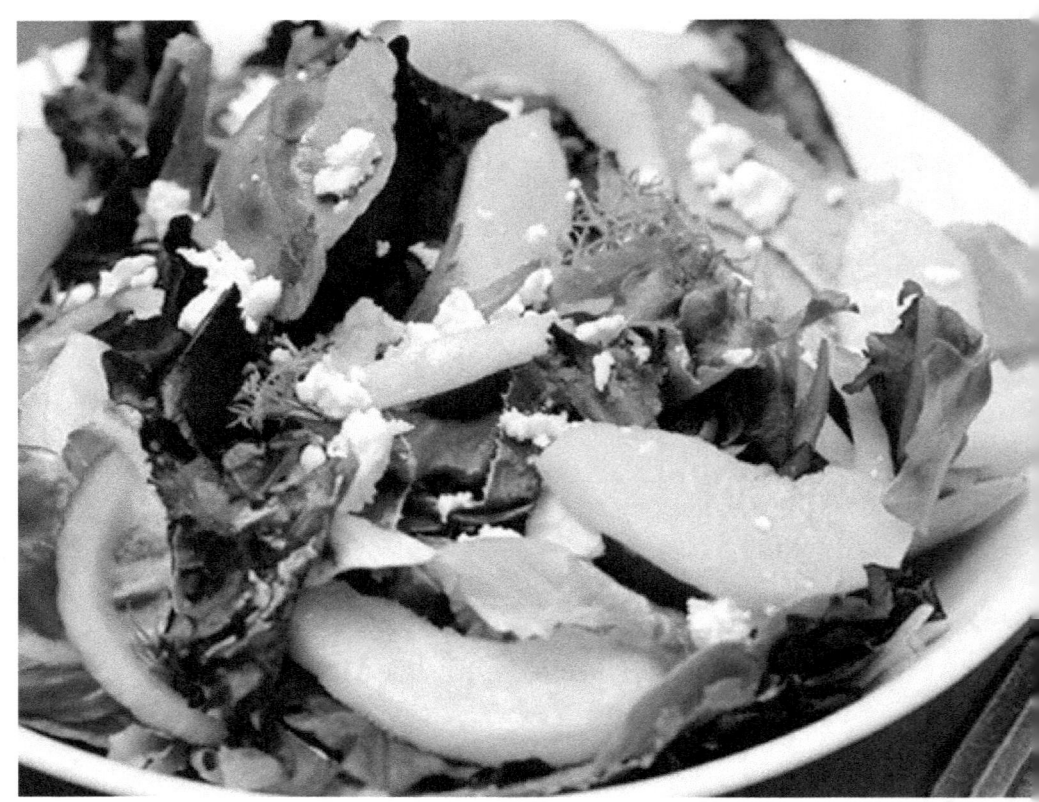

Nutritional Value:

Calories: 108

Total fat: 0g

Sat. fat: 0g

Trans. Fat: 0g

Cholesterol: 5mg

Sodium: 430mg

Carbs: 25g

Fiber: 5g

Sugar: 10g

Protein: 5g

Title: Chicken, Lemon & Oil Salad- a quick-fix for a packed lunch, it is easy to prepare, carry and eat while outside the comforts of home.

Servings: 2

Ingredients:

1 cup spinach, torn

½ avocado, peeled, seeded and chopped

1/3 red onion

½ cucumber, sliced

8 almonds, halved

1 carrot, grated

1 cup bean sprouts

1 tomato, diced

½ cup parsley

1 cup chopped chicken breast

For the dressing: 1 lemon, juiced 1 tsp extra virgin olive oil, 1tsp oregano salt and pepper to taste

Directions:

Toss all ingredients in a large bowl

In a separate bowl, whisk dressing ingredients and drizzle on mixture

Serve

Picture:

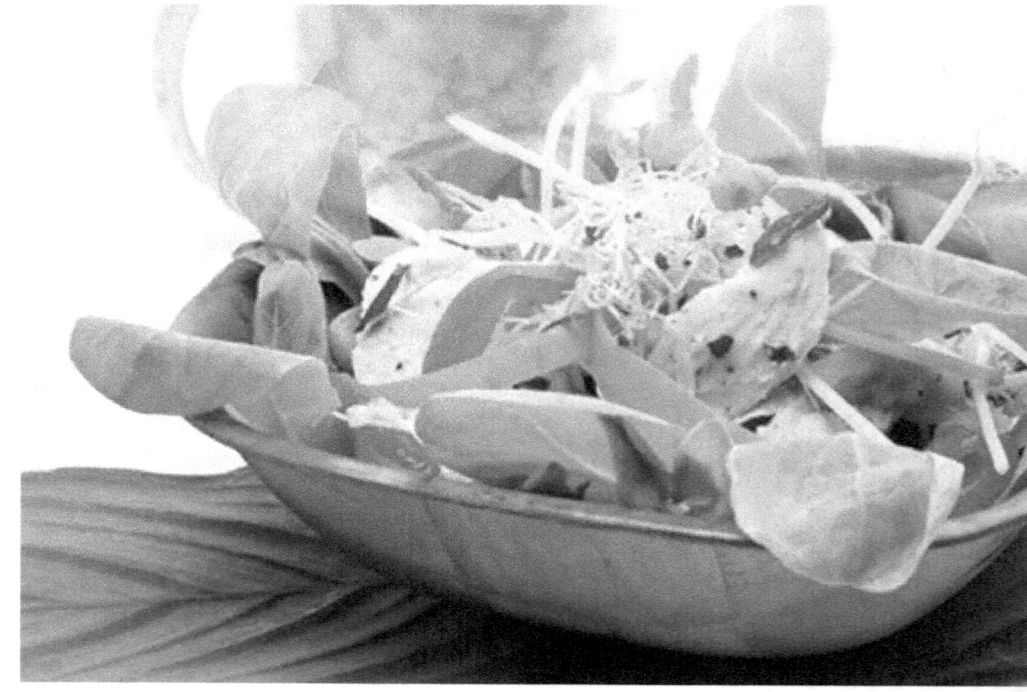

Nutritional Value:

Calories: 220

Total fat: 17g

Sat. fat: 2.3g

Trans fat: 0g

Cholesterol: 0mg

Sodium: 49mg

Carbs: 16g

Fiver: 8g

Sugar: 4g

Protein: 5g

Title: Quinoa Salad: a complete meal that will be the delight of vegetarians, it contains all essential nutrients with only veggie based ingredients.

Servings: 8

Ingredients:

1 cup quinoa

½ cup chopped white onion

1 tsp extra virgin olive oil

2 cups water

1 orange

¼ cup pecans, chopped and toasted

2 tbsp minced red onion

5 dates, pitted and chopped

½ lb asparagus

½ peppers diced

For the dressing: 2tbsp lemon juice, 1tbsp extra virgin olive oil, 1 clove garlic, minced 2 tbsp mint, chopped ¼ tsp salt and pepper

Directions:

Heat skillet on low and put oil and onion, cook for 2 minutes

Add quinoa and cook for 5 minutes

Add water and salt and allow boiling

Cover and let simmer for 15 minutes

Remove from heat and wait for 15 minutes

Put mixture on bowl and remaining ingredients, toss

In a separate bowl, whisk juice and remaining ingredients

Pour dressing on mixture and garnish with mint

Serve

Picture:

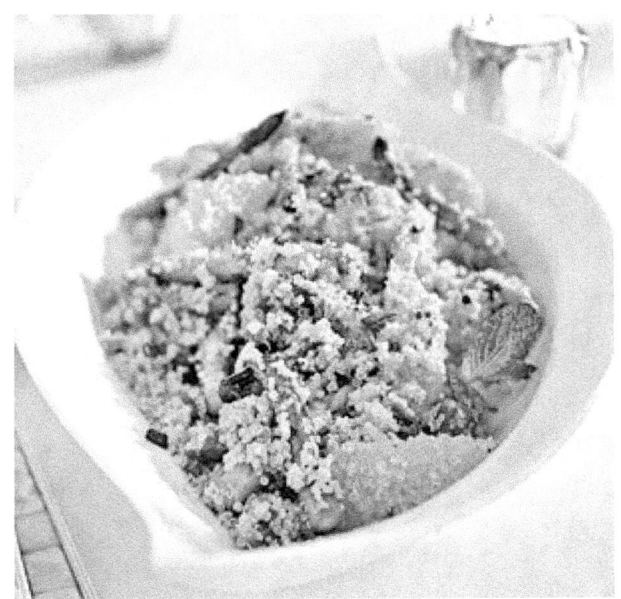

Nutritional Value:

Calories: 164

Fat: 6g

Sat. fat: 1g

Sodium: 186mg

Carbs: 25g

Cholesterol: 0mg

Fiber: 4g

Protein: 5g

Title: Steaks in Marmalade- a Clean Eating treat packed with your dose of protein for the day, the sweetness of the side will balance the taste of the steak.

Servings: 4

Ingredients:

4 beef steaks, trimmed

1 red onion, cut into rings

2 tbsp honey

2 tbsp red wine vinegar

1 tsp thyme

Sea salt and pepper

Directions:

Heat broiler

In a skillet on medium heat, coat with cooking spray

Add onion, cover and cook for 3 minutes

Add salt, honey and vinegar

Remove cover and simmer for 8 minutes, stir occasionally

On the beef, sprinkle salt, thyme and pepper evenly

Put beef of broiler and broil for 4 minutes on each side

Garnish with mixture

Serve

Picture:

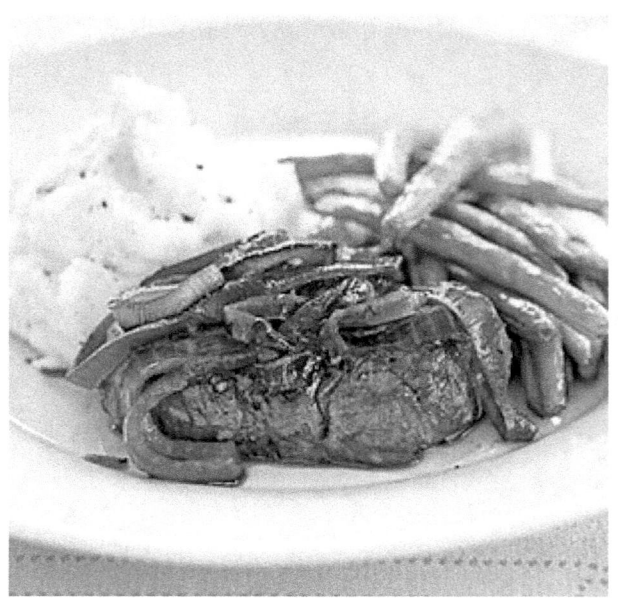

Nutritional Value:

Calories: 289

Total fat: 12g

Carbs: 12g

Fiber: 1g

Cholesterol: 95mg

Sodium: 369mg

Protein: 33g

Title: Crab Salad- a simple but challenging dish to prepare but its reward in terms of taste, texture and nutrients will more than make up for it.

Servings: 8

Ingredients:

1 cup crabmeat

3 tbsp Greek yogurt

2 tbsp extra virgin olive oil

8 eggs, boiled, peeled and halved

1 tbsp lemon juice

2 cups sliced radishes

24 lettuce leaves

1 tsp Dijon mustard

¼ cup celery

Sea salt and pepper

Directions:

In a separate bowl, toss radish, juice and salt, cover and put on fridge for 30 minutes

Remove egg yolks and combine with juice, salt and pepper in a separate bowl, whisk while adding oil

Add yogurt in mixture, then crabmeat, mustard and celery, stir gently

Spread lettuce leaves and top with egg whites

Add crabmeat mixture on top

Put radish mixture on side

Serve

Picture:

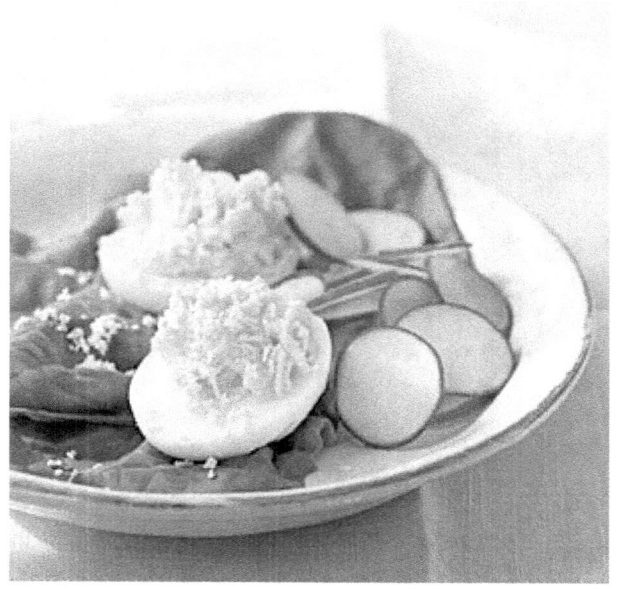

Nutritional Value:

Calories: 140

Total fat: 9g

Sat. fat: 2g

Carbs: 4g

Fiber: 2g

Cholesterol: 230mg

Sodium: 400mg

Protein: 12g

10 Dinners

Title: Stuffed Sweet Potatoes- a colorful and interesting dish to prepare, its presentation is a match to its healthy contents.

Servings: 4

Ingredients:

4 sweet potatoes

1 cup chopped tomatoes

1 tsp olive oil

1 clove minced garlic

1 red diced onion

1 tsp ground cumin

½ tsp chili flakes

½ cup cooked black beans

2 tbsp chopped cilantro

Sea salt and pepper to taste

Directions:

Heat oven to 400 degrees

Put sweet potatoes on baking sheet

Bake for 30 minutes

Prick with a few and bake for another 30 minutes

Heat skillet on medium heat

Add oil and onions and cook for 2 minutes

Add garlic and cook until golden brown

Add cumin, chili, salt, tomatoes and bean.

Add cilantro and salt and pepper to taste

Halve potatoes and top with mixture

Serve

Picture:

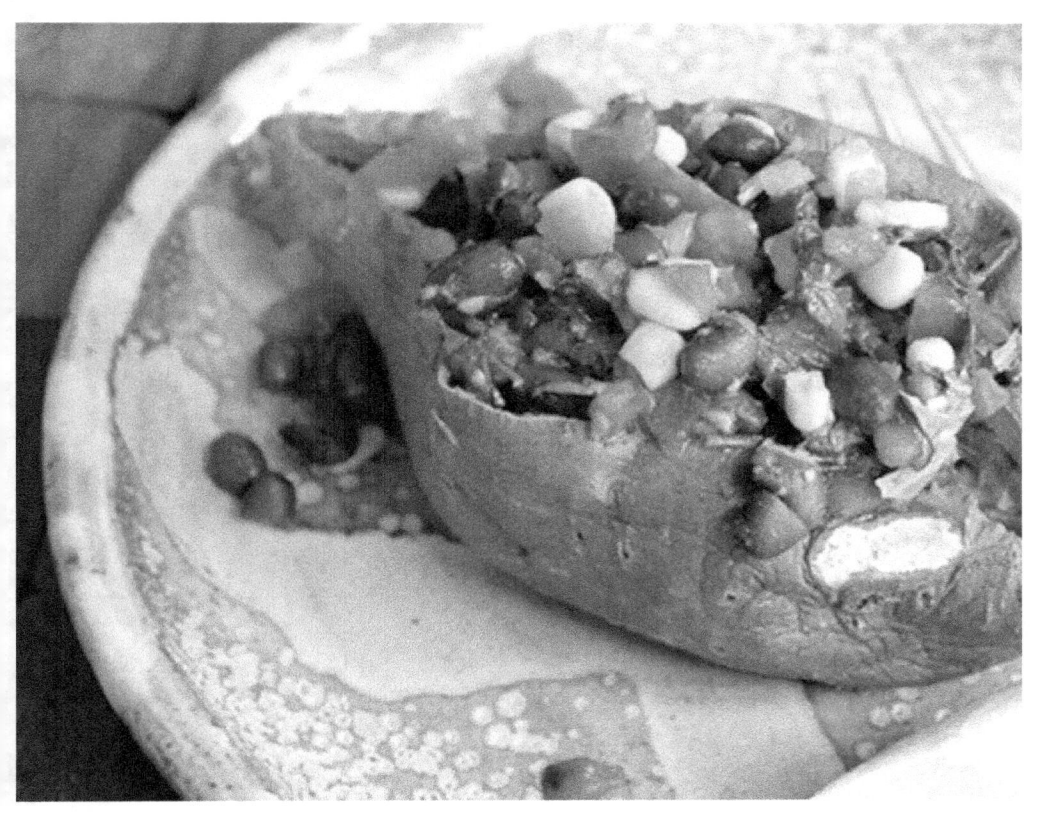

Nutritional Value:

Calories: 215

Total fat: 2g

Sat. fat: 1g

Trans fat: 0g

Cholesterol: 0g

Sodium: 15mg

Carbs: 43g

Fiber: 8g

Sugar: 3.5g

Protein: 8.5g

Title: Brussels sprouts Salad- a lazy dinner for a lazy evening, easy to prepare but filled with flavor and nutrients.

Servings: 6

Ingredients:

1 lb Brussels sprouts, halved

2 tsp extra virgin oil

1 clove garlic, minced

2 tbsp walnuts, chopped and toasted

½ oz. Asiago cheese

1/3 cup breadcrumbs

Sea salt and pepper

Directions:

Heat skillet on medium heat, add 1 tsp oil and garlic, cook for 1 minute

Add crumbs and cook for 1 minute

Remove and set aside on a bowl

Add oil on skillet and add separated leaves of sprouts, cook for 8 minutes

Toss with mixture and add salt and pepper

Top with nuts and cheese

Serve

Picture:

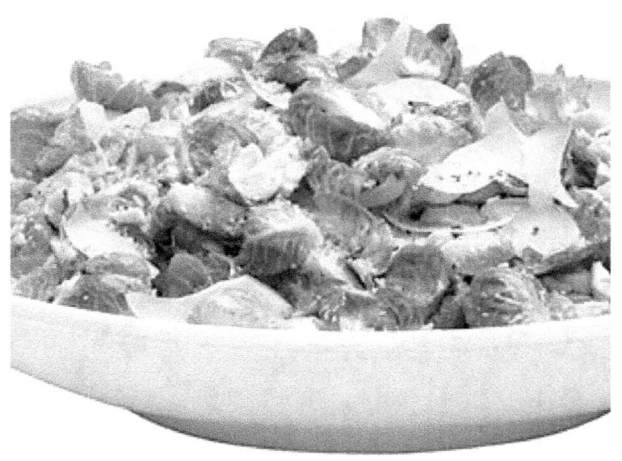

Nutritional Value:

Calories: 71

Total fat: 3g

Sat. fat: 1g

Carbs: 9g

Fiber: 2g

Cholesterol: 1mg

Sodium: 160mg

Protein: 4g

Title: Glazed Salmon- a great way to treat yourself with a hearty meal and the familiar comfort of sweet salmon.

Servings: 2

Ingredients:

8 oz salmon fillet

1 tbsp Dijon mustard

1 tbsp honey

1 tbsp lemon juice

Salt and pepper

Directions:

Heat oven to broil

In a separate bowl, whisk juice, mustard and honey

In a baking sheet, spread the salmon. Drizzle with mixture on both sides

Broil for 5 minutes on each side

Serve

Picture:

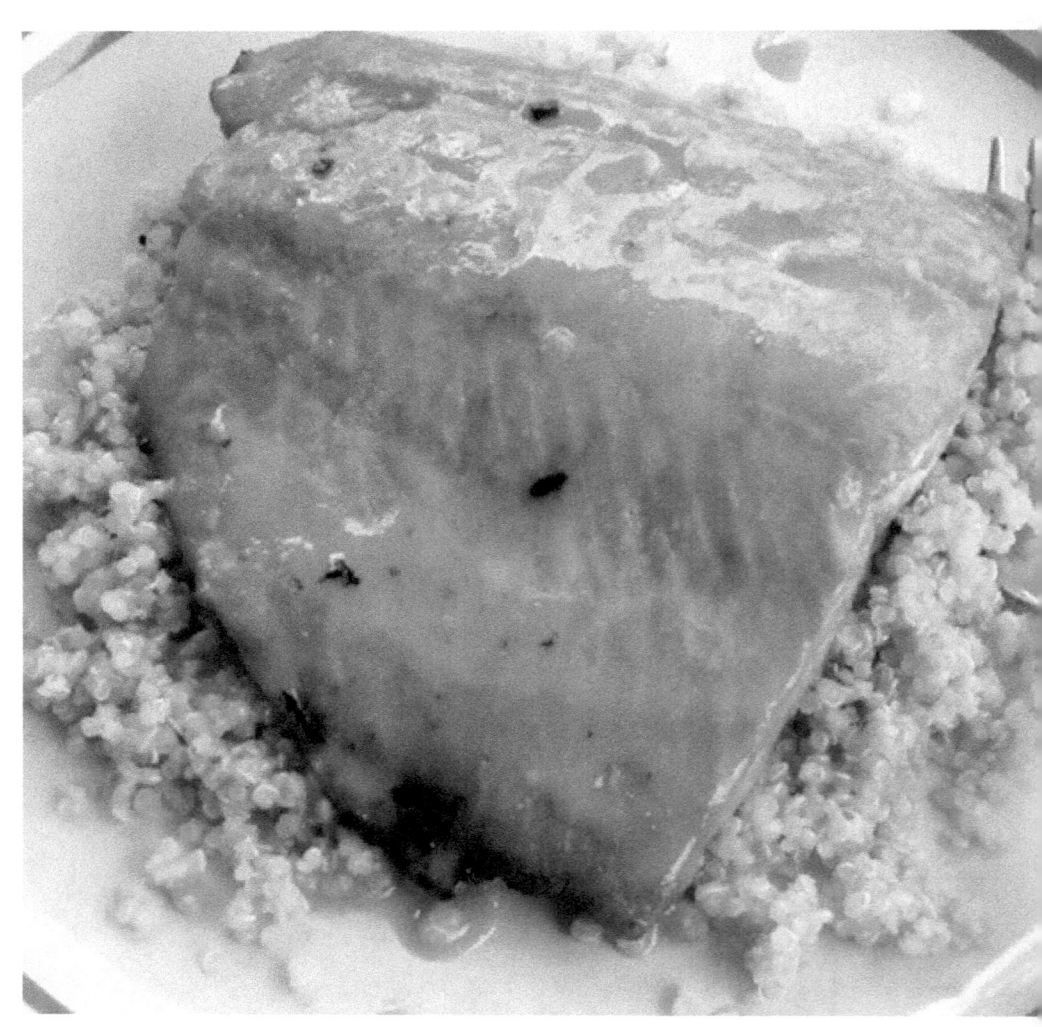

Nutritional Value:

Calories: 245

Total fat: 9g

Sat. fat: 1g

Trans fat: 0g

Cholesterol: 80 mg

Sodium: 126mg

Carbs: 9g

Fiber: 0g

Protein: 29g

Title: Lasagna Rolls- a healthy version of a favorite, mimic the taste without sacrificing the lifestyle.

Servings: 5

Ingredients:

5 whole wheat lasagna noodles, cooked to al dente and drained

½ jar unsweetened marinara sauce

2 cloves garlic, minced

1 tbsp olive oil

1 cup low fat ricotta cheese

6 cups spinach, chopped

1.5 cup skim mozzarella, shredded

½ cup low fat cottage cheese

1 egg white

¼ cup parmesan, grated

Sea salt and pepper

Directions:

Heat oven to 425 degrees

Put marinara to casserole dish

In a skillet, heat to low and add oil and garlic for 1 minute

Add spinach and cook for 3 minutes

In a separate bowl, toss mixture with remaining ingredients

In a flat surface, ¼ cup of mixture on each of the noodles

Sprinkle with remaining cheese

Put noodles on casserole and cover with foil

Bake for 20 minutes

Serve

Picture:

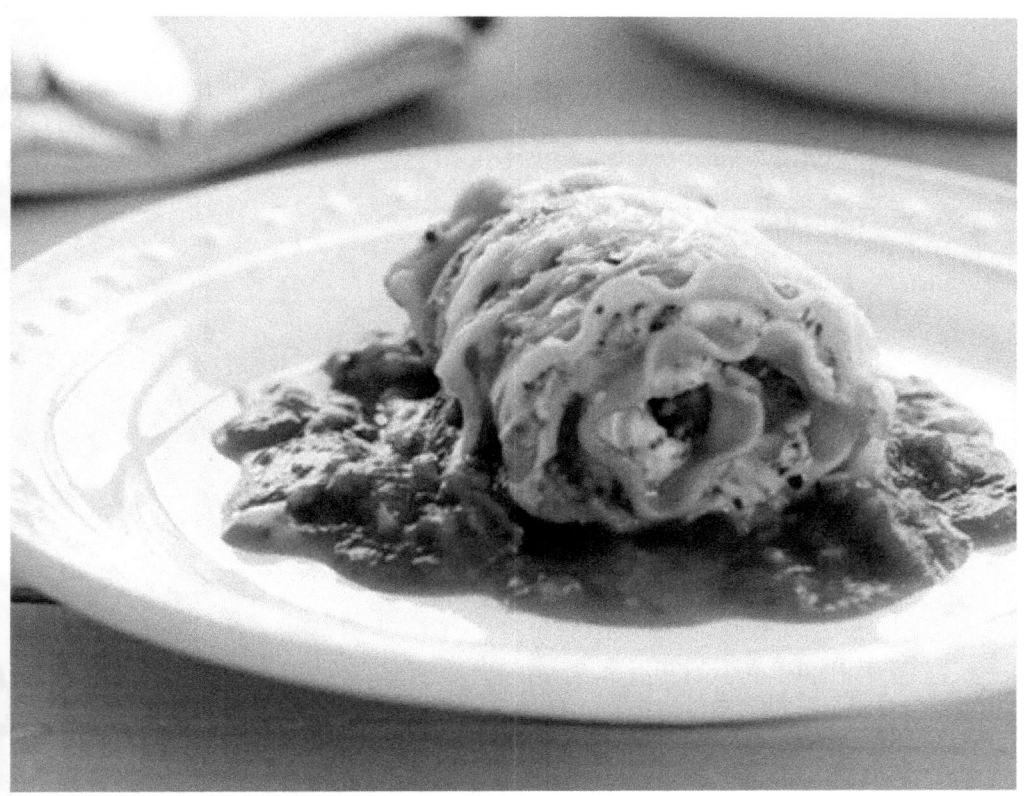

Nutritional Value:

Calories: 240

Total fat: 9g

Sat. fat: 4g

Cholesterol: 18g

Carbs: 25g

Fiber: 5g

Sugar: 4g

Sodium: 460mg

Protein: 15g

Title: Fish & Rice: a healthy and heavy dinner for a long evening ahead, it is packed with nutrients that can energize especially for when you need it the most.

Servings: 6

Ingredients:

1.5 lbs any white fish fillet cut into 1 in. squares

1 tbsp lemon juice

½ cup Greek yogurt

2 tbsp extra virgin olive oil

2 cloves garlic

1 cup long brown rice

½ cup onion, diced

1 cup tomatoes, diced

1 cup low sodium, fat free vegetable broth

1 tsp capers

½ tsp red pepper

1 tbsp thyme

Salt and pepper

Directions:

In a separate bowl, whisk juice and yogurt

Add fish and coat with mixture

Leave at refrigerator

Cook rice by adding oil to skillet

Heat to low and add onion and garlic, cook for 5 minutes

Add rice and rest of ingredients, stir

Cover for 40 minutes

Add fish and cook for 10 minutes

Serve

Picture:

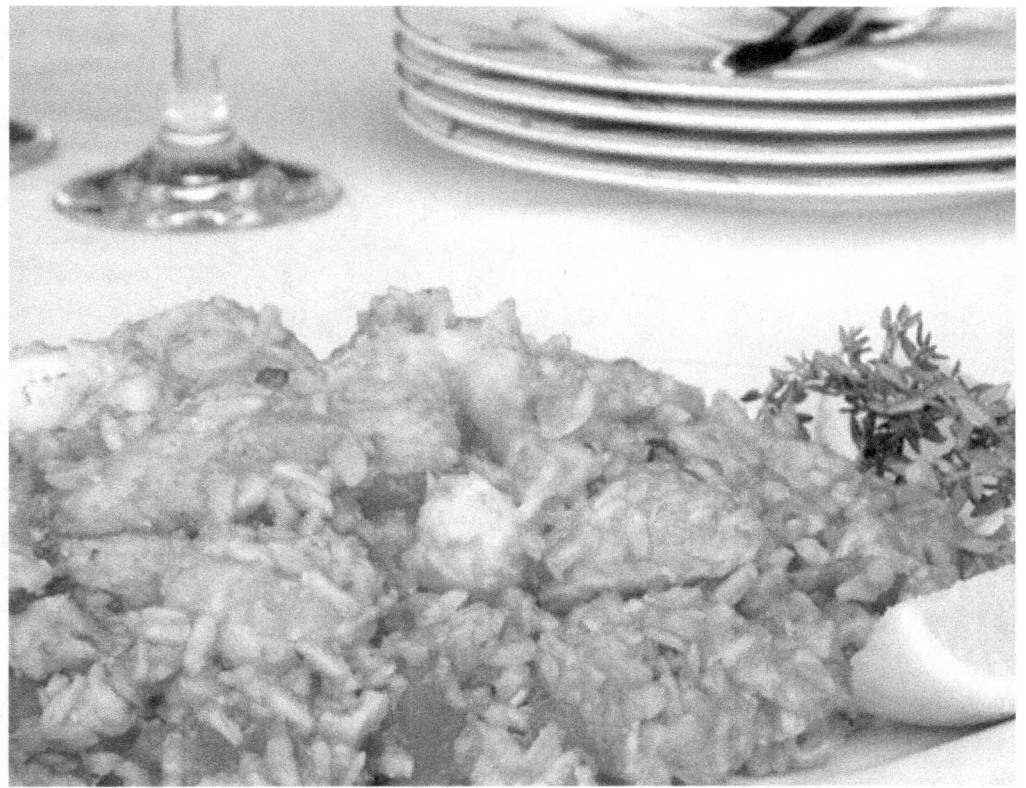

Nutritional Value:

Calories: 150

Total fat: 5g

Sat. fat: 1g

Trans fat: 0g

Cholesterol: 17mg

Sodium: 125mg

Carbs: 14g

Fiber: 2g

Sugar: 3g

Protein: 11g

Title: Herb Pasta- a perfect balance of nutritional requirements that can be a joy to prepare and to eat.

Servings: 8

Ingredients:

1 13oz. whole wheat pasta, spaghetti or linguine

2 cloves garlic, minced

¼ cup extra virgin olive oil

1 tbsp basil, chopped

1 tbsp caper

1 tbsp thyme

1 tbsp parsley

¼ tsp red pepper flakes

2 cups arugula

2 cup tomatoes, sliced

Sea salt and pepper

Directions:

In a skillet on low heat, add oil and garlic, cook for 1 minute

Add salt and pepper, herbs and capers, cook for 1 minute

Add cooked pasta and arugula, toss

Cook until arugula wilts and remove from heat

Add tomatoes

Serve

Picture:

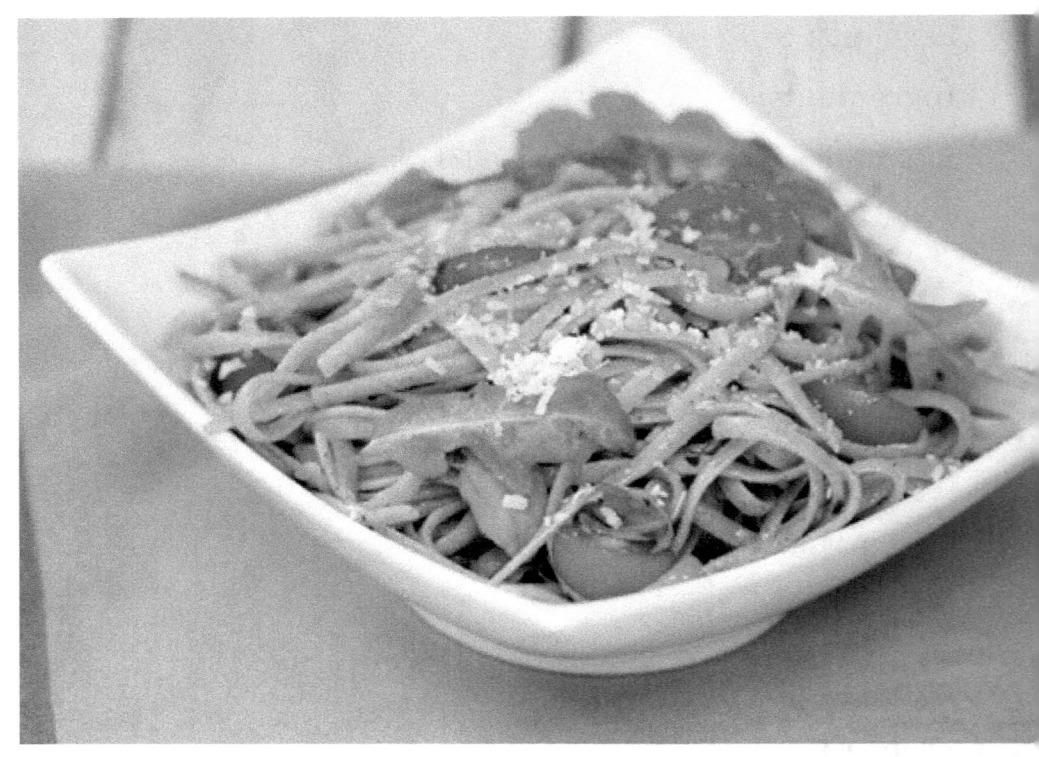

Nutritional Value:

Calories: 126

Total fat: 7g

Sat. fat: 1g

Trans fat: 0g

Cholesterol: 0mg

Sodium: 35mg

Carbs: 13g

Fiber: 2g

Sugar: 2g

Protein: 2g

Title: Mediterranean Chicken: another challenging recipe but can provide a delightful change from the usual chicken recipes.

Servings: 4

Ingredients:

4 chicken breasts, deboned and skinned

1 tbsp basil

2 tbsp olives

¼ cup feta cheese

1 red bell pepper, halved

Directions:

Heat broiler

Put peppers on baking sheet and broil for 15 minutes

Put in zipped bag and seal for 15 minutes

Open, peel and chop

Heat grill to medium

Toss pepper, cheese, basil and olives

Cut slit on chicken to form a pocket and stuff with mixture

Season chicken with salt and pepper

Grill chicken for 6 minutes on each side

Picture:

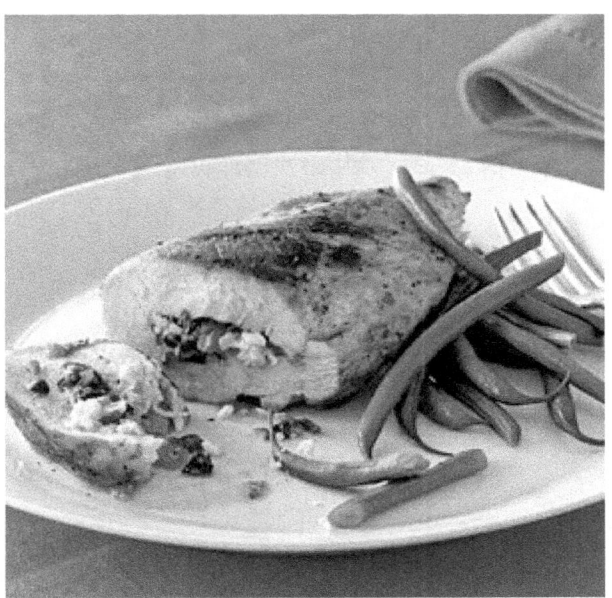

Nutritional Value:

Calories: 210

Total fat: 6g

Sat fat: 2g

Carbs: 2g

Fiber: 1g

Cholesterol: 98mg

Sodium: 266mg

Protein: 35g

Title: Tuna with Herb Topping- looks difficult to make but actually easy to prepare, it is a balance of acid, sweetness and saltiness.

Servings: 4

Ingredients:

4 tuna steaks, halved

¼ cup almonds, chopped

¼ cup tangerine juice

1tbsp extra virgin olive oil

2 tbsp chopped red onion

2 tbsp chopped mint

½ tsp chopped fennel seeds

Salt and pepper

Directions:

In a separate bowl, combine almonds, onions, mint, juice, seeds and oil

Sprinkle salt and pepper on top of fish

Heat skillet on medium and coat with oil

Add fish and cook for 1 minute on each side

Remove fish and drizzle with mixture

Serve

Picture:

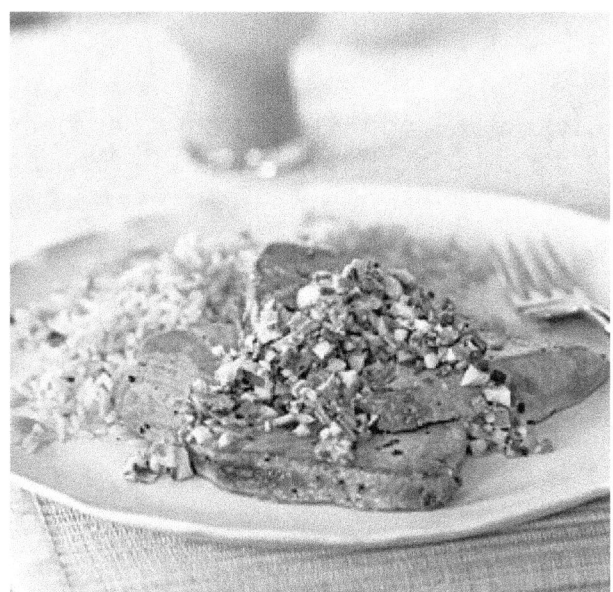

Nutritional Value:

Calories: 277

Total fat: 10 g

Sat. fat: 1g

Carbs: 4g

Fiber: 1g

Cholesterol: 77mg

Sodium: 350mg

Protein: 42g

Title: Balsamic Chicken: a loading of protein when daily consumption does not meet its target, the burst of flavors can make any dinner interesting.

Servings: 5

Ingredients:

3 chicken breasts, deboned and skinned

1 cup of tomatoes, sliced

2 cloves garlic

¼ cup balsamic vinegar

1tbsp olive oil

1 tsp oregano, rosemary and basil

¼ tsp thyme

Salt and pepper

Directions:

In a slow cooker, pour oil on bottom

Sprinkle salt and pepper into chicken

Add chicken in cooker

Put onions on top and then all herbs and garlic

Pour vinegar and add tomatoes

Cook on high for 4 hours

Picture:

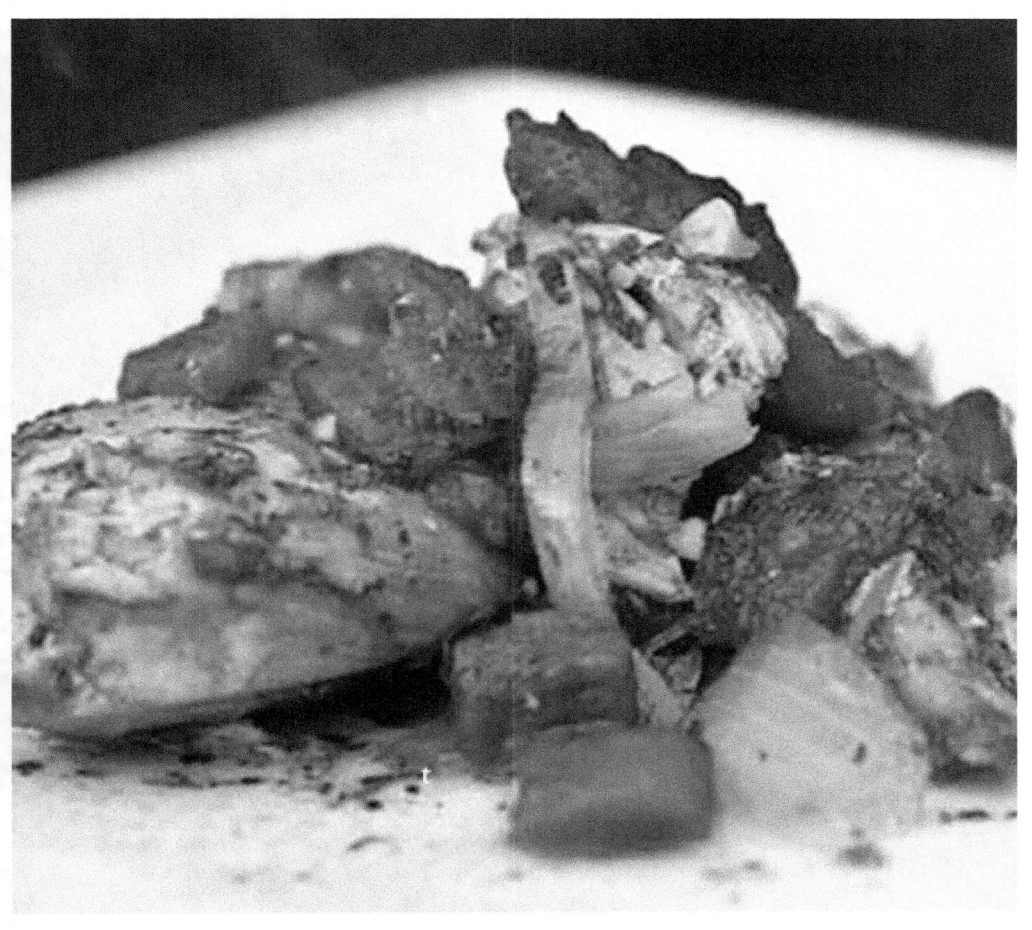

Nutritional Value:

Calories: 190

Total Fat: 6g

Sat. fat: 1g

Trans fat: 0g

Cholesterol: 53mg

Sodium: 121mg

Carbs: 5g

Fiber: 1g

Sugar: 3g

Protein: 26g

Title: Fajitas- another healthy version of a comfort food, perfect recipe to start or cap an evening.

Servings: 4

Ingredients:

4 leaves lettuce

2 whole wheat pita pockets

2 tsp oregano

4 oz. white mushrooms, sliced

1 lb beef sirloin, cut into thin strips

1 red bell pepper, cut into strips

2 cloves garlic, minced

1 red onion, cut into strips

2 tbsp olive oil

Directions:

Heat oven to 350 degrees

In a skillet on low heat, sauté mushrooms in oil for 6 minutes

Add pepper, garlic and onion and cook for 4 minutes

Add beef and cook for 10 minutes

Sprinkle with oregano, salt and pepper

Cover and simmer for 5 minutes then drain

Cut pita in half and brush with oil

Put in baking sheet and put in oven for 5 minutes

Put mixture into pita pockets and add lettuce

Serve

Picture:

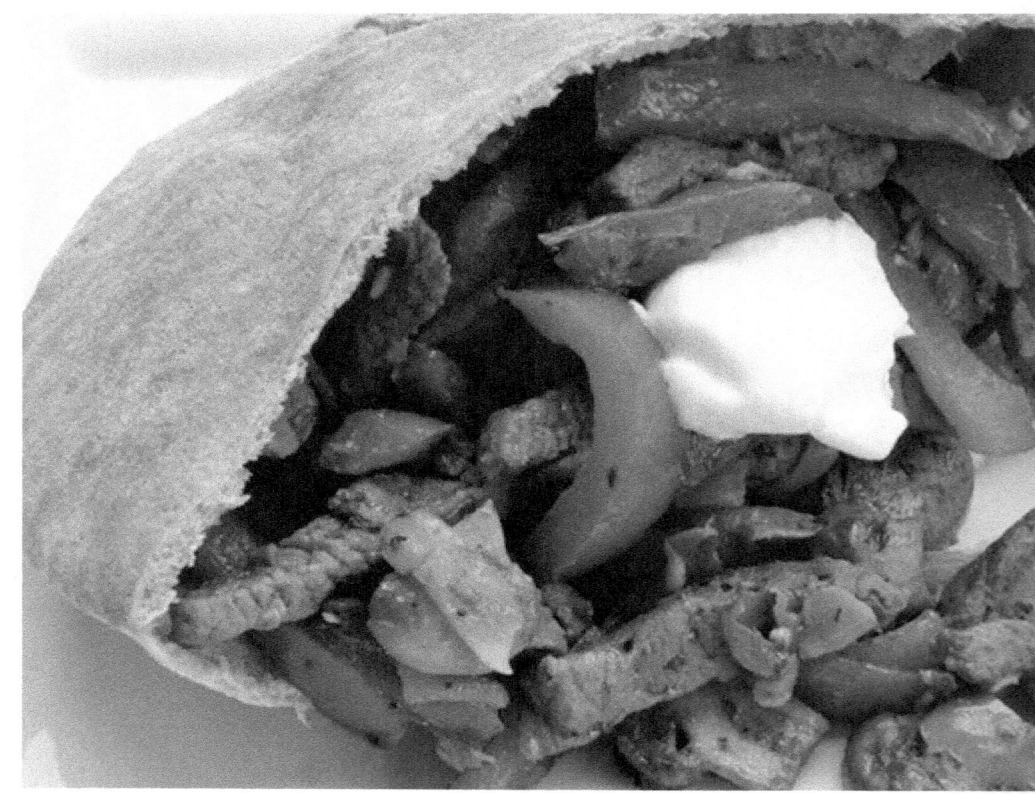

Nutritional Value:

Calories: 255

Total fat: 6g

Sat. fat: 2g

Trans fat: 0g

Cholesterol: 70mg

Sodium: 235mg

Carbs: 21g

Fiber: 3g

Sugar: 2g

Protein: 29g

5 Snacks

Title: Berry Parfait- a perfect snack to prepare for the weekend, it is a flexible recipe that can allow changes in main fruits.

Servings: 4

Ingredients:

1 cup oats

½ tsp cinnamon

½ cup almonds, sliced

3 tbsp unrefined coconut oil

½ cup each of raspberries, blueberries and blackberries

2 cups of Greek yogurt

Directions:

Heat oven to 350 degrees

In a separate bowl, combine cinnamon, almonds and oats

Stir with oil

Spread mixture on baking sheet

Bake for 20 minutes

Top with berries

Picture:

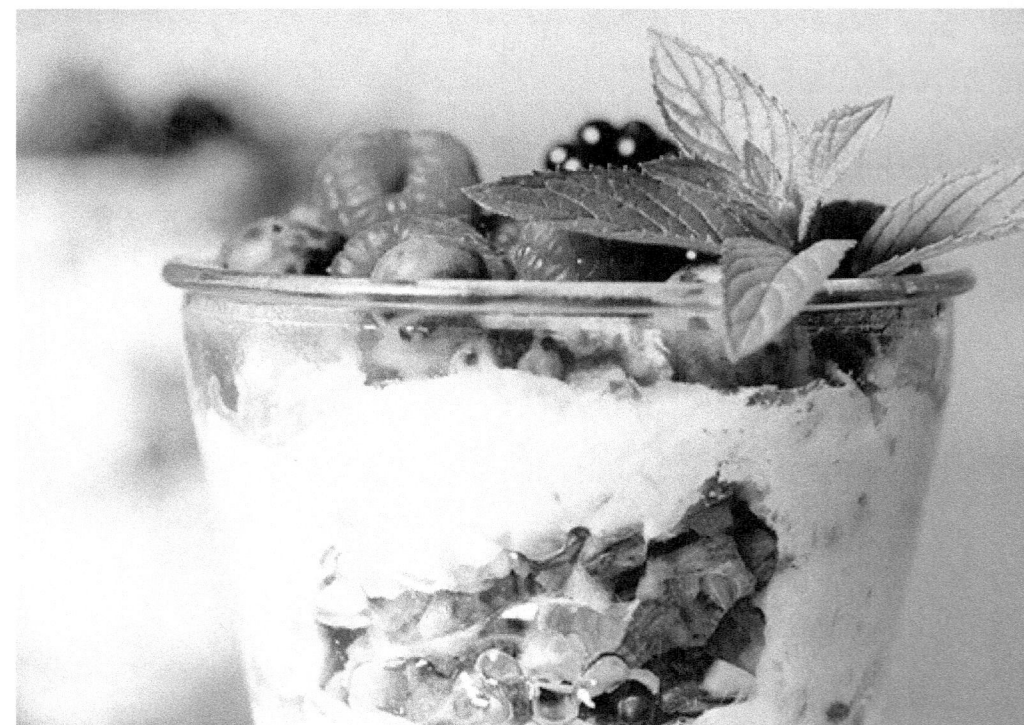

Nutritional Value:

Calories: 139

Total fat: 1g

Sat. fat: 0g

Trans fat: 0g

Cholesterol: 2mg

Sodium: 32mg

Carbs: 26g

Fiber: 5g

Sugar: 17g

Protein: 8g

Title: Homemade Peanut Butter- a guilt-free healthy alternative that can enhance future meals and snacks.

Servings: 8 oz.

Ingredients:

3 cups raw peanuts, shelled

½ tsp sea salt

Directions:

Heat oven to 350 degrees

Spread nuts on a baking sheet and roast for 20 minutes

Stir occasionally and cool for 10 minutes

Put peanuts on food processor

Sprinkle and process for 10 minutes

When buttery or smooth remove and keep in glass jar

Refrigerate

Picture:

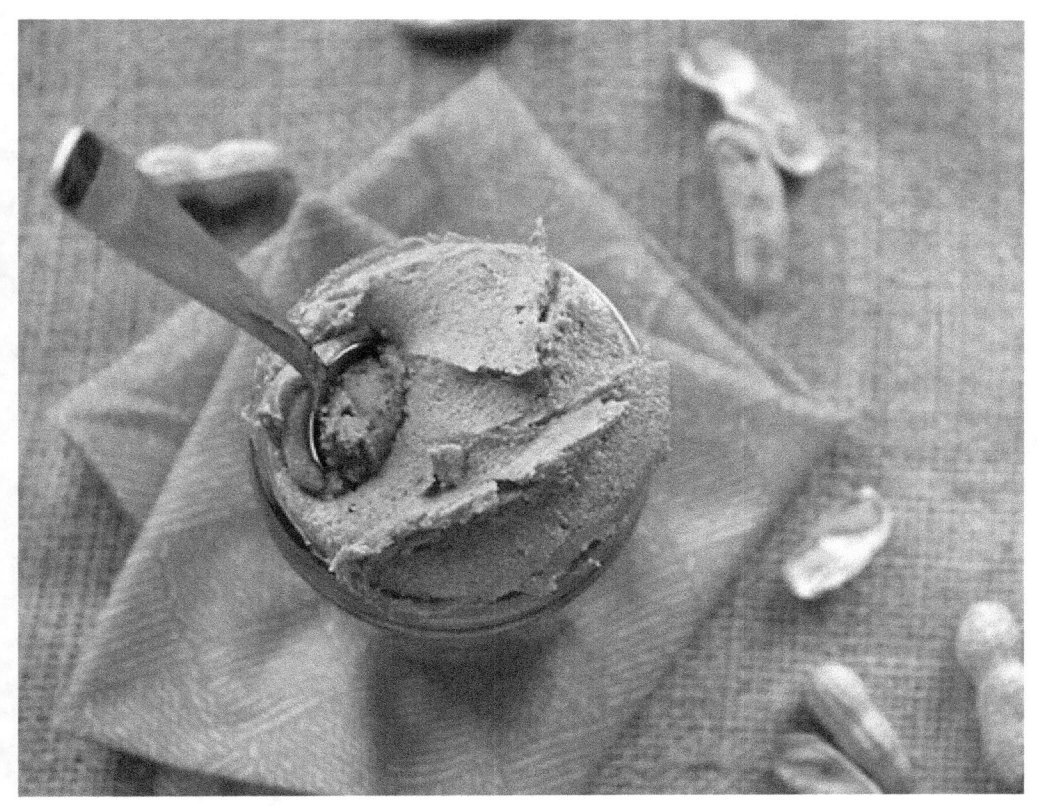

Nutritional Value:

Calories: 166

Total fat: 15g

Sat. fat: 2g

Trans fat: 0g

Cholesterol: 0g

Sodium: 70mg

Carbs: 5mg

Fiber: 3g

Sugar: 1g

Protein: 8g

Title: Pecans- a snack that can be prepared in bulk and packed for outings or consumed on a quiet afternoon.

Servings: 8

Ingredients:

1 lb raw pecans, halved

2 tbsp honey

½ tsp onion powder

¼ tsp garlic powder

½ tsp cayenne pepper

Directions:

In a slow cooker, combine all ingredients, coat pecans with honey and the spices

Cover and cook for 15 minutes on high

Change to low and cook for 1 hour, stir occasionally

Cool and store in airtight container

Picture:

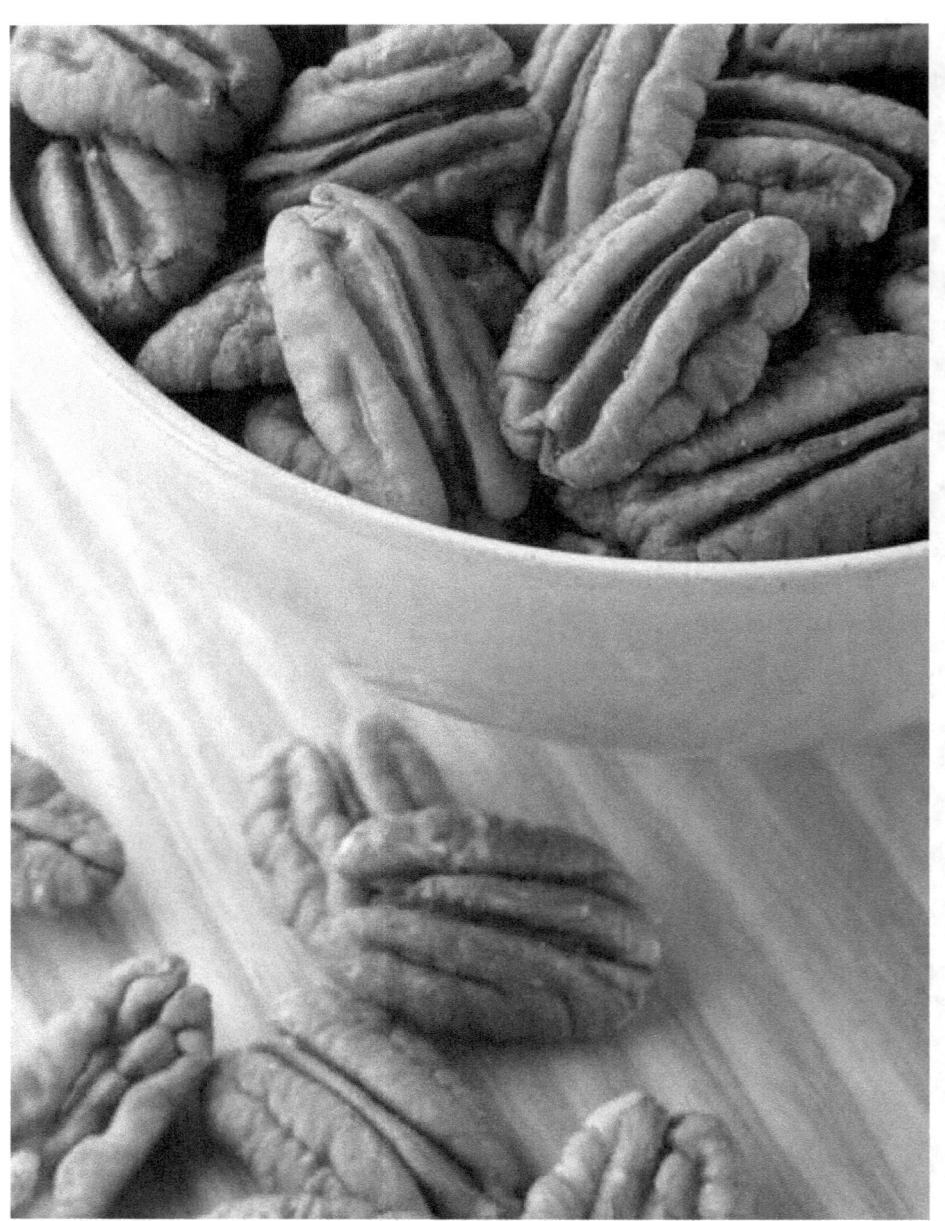

Nutritional Value:

Calories 218

Total fat: 20g

Sat. fat: 2g

Trans fat: 0g

Cholesterol: 0g

Sodium: 5g

Carbs: 12g

Fiber: 3g

Sugar: 9g

Protein: 3g

Title: Potato Crunch- a snack that can either be eaten by itself or used as a side or ingredients for other main courses.

Servings: 2

Ingredients:

1 sweet potato, peeled and julienned

1 tbsp olive oil

Salt and pepper

Directions:

Heat oven to 375 degrees

In a separate bowl, add potato strings, salt and pepper and drizzle with oil, toss

Spread strings on baking sheet

Bake for30 minutes

Store in airtight container

Picture:

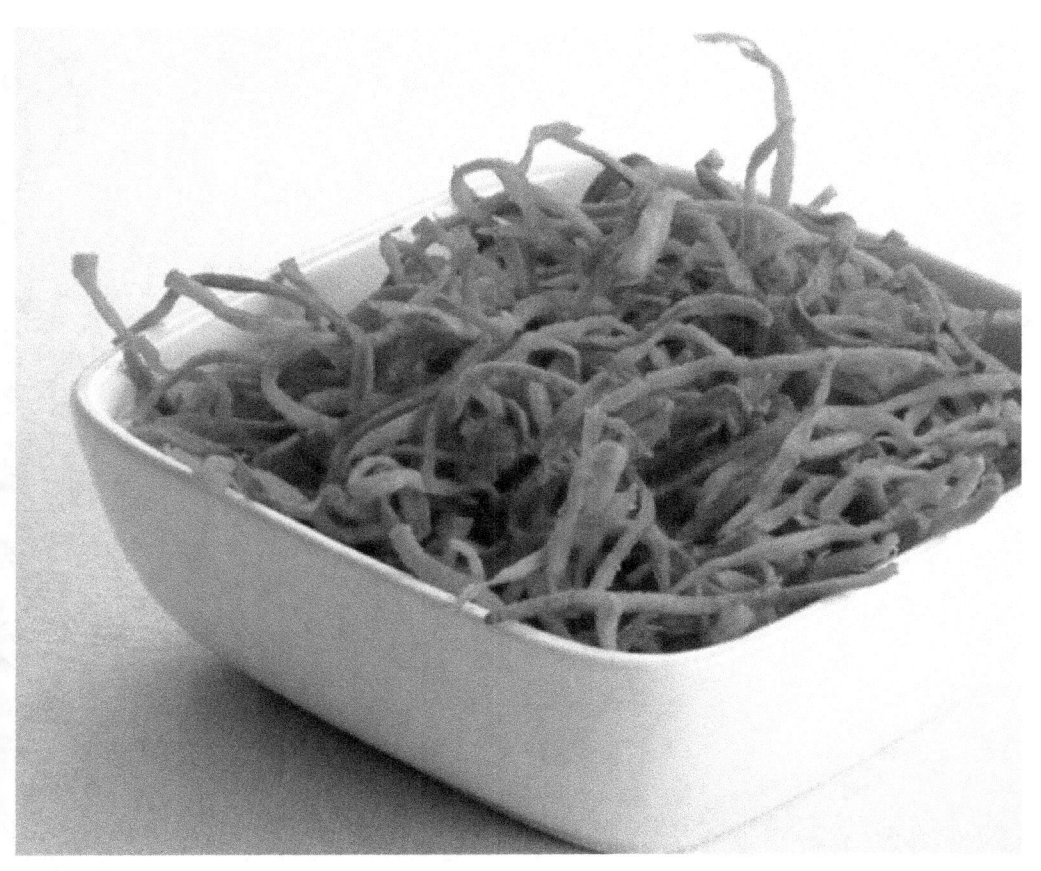

Nutritional Value:

Calories: 117

Total fat: 7g

Sat. fat: 1g

Trans fat: 0g

Carbs: 13g

Sodium: 210mg

Fiber: 2g

Sugar: 4g

Protein: 1g

Title: Smoothie- a perfect snack before or after a workout or a busy and tiring day, it is refreshing and healthy at the same time.

Servings: 3

Ingredients:

1 cup crushed ice

½ cup pomegranate juice

1 cup unsweetened green tea

½ cup Greek yogurt

1 cup blueberries

1 banana, sliced

1 cup spinach

½ slice ginger

Directions:

In a blender, put all ingredients and blend till smooth

Serve cold

Picture:

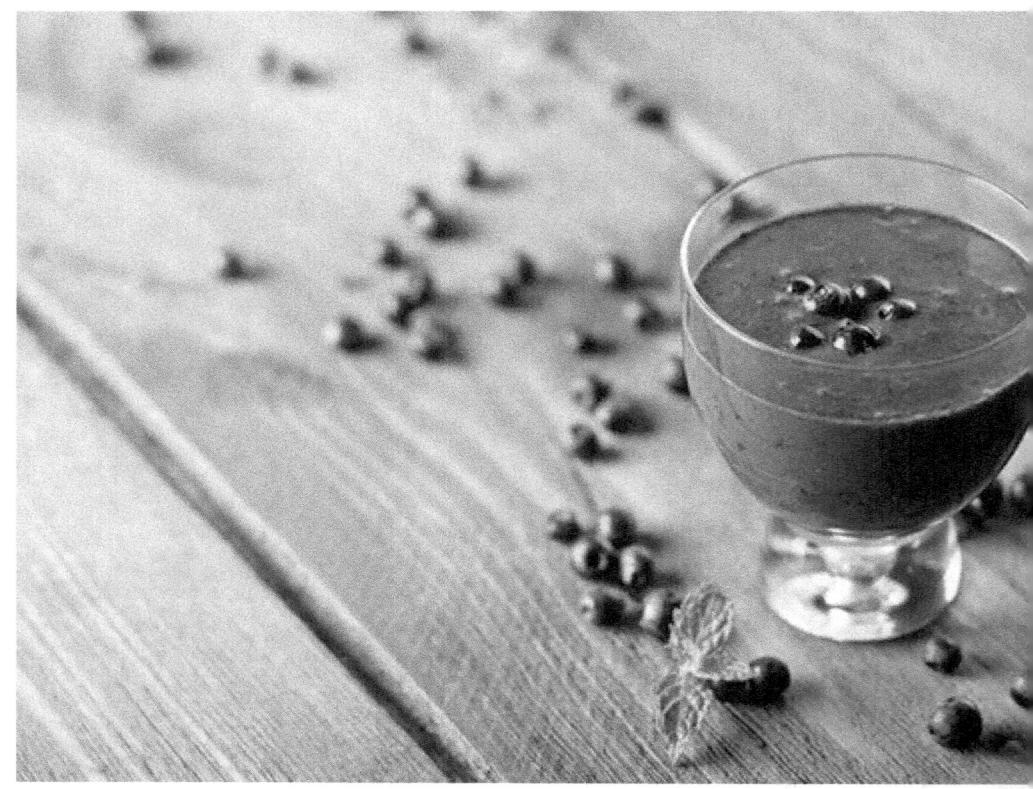

Nutritional Value:

Calories: 131

Total fat: 1g

Sat. fat: 0g

Trans fat: 0g

Cholesterol: 2mg

Sodium: 287mg

Carbs: 26g

Fiber: 4g

Sugar: 13g

Protein: 7g

Conclusion

Clean Eating is one of the best health and lifestyle decisions that you will make. With its wide range of benefits, from weight loss, energy gain, protection from diseases and savings on finances, Clean Eating is becoming the lifestyle of choice.

I hope this guide was able to provide you with a working knowledge on the basics of Clean Eating, its principles, preparation and recommendations. To start with your new lifestyle, take a look at your kitchen and begin to be critical with the contents. Take note of the processed foods and find out the substitutes on your next trip to the grocery.

Once you are ready, begin to cook at home with Clean Eating-friendly food items and discover how this lifestyle allows you to eat healthy foods without sacrificing taste and flavor.

Remember, a Clean Eating lifestyle is not a fantasy that you could only dream of but it is a reality that you can truly fulfill.